IOWA'S EARLY HOME REMEDIES

by

Armstrong, Erin
Ball, Jarett
Brown, Stephen
Bryant, Daniel
Cross, Jason
Foor, Ryan
Gerst, Bobby
Hagele, Matt
Hagele, Mike
Heater, Jaime
Hodges, Bob
Hollingsworth, Les
Housman, Crystal
Lanz, Denise
Locke, Aaron
Lowe, Travis
Newman, Nathan
Reighard, Anna
Samuels, Tina
Scott, Buddy
Simmons, Nicole
Spitznogle, Erin
Stone, Seth
Whipple, Allison
Whipple, Lindsey
Young, Anna
Young, Mrs.

QUIXOTE PRESS
R.R. #4, Box 33B
Blvd. Station
Sioux City, Iowa 51109

Printed
For
Quixote Press
by
BRENNAN PRINTING
100 Main Street
Deep River, Iowa 52222
515-595-2000

* * * * * * * * * *

QUIXOTE
PRESS
Bruce Carlson
R.R. *#4, Box 33B*
Blvd. Station
Sioux City, Iowa
51109

PRINTED IN U.S.A.

DEDICATION

. . . to our inventive grandparents.

Table of Contents

INTRODUCTION

This book is a collection of remedies that families used back in the days when doctors were not sent for unless there was an extreme emergency and the drugstore was a rarity. It was a time when oranges were only for the wealthy and a hospital only if you were near death. Money was tight. A person learned to make do with what they had. Mothers often became doctor and pharmacist.

Collecting these creative remedies seemed an appropriate task for some creative students. These students are members of an enrichment class at Wapello Elementary School in Wapello, Iowa.

The students rediscovered these remedies from grandparents, aunts, and uncles, and other helpful people in the state. We must thank the whole Wapello-Oakville community for the key role in this project.

It is interesting to ponder why or how some of these remedies worked. It is also interesting and understandable how several remedies, or the ingredients, are repeated. If a remedy appeared to help, it would have been shared to help others.

We hope, as you read these remedies, you will remember back to different times; times of struggle and times of self-reliance. And we can all try to understand what life was like then.

Beth Young
Teacher

The reader is warned that these remedies have **not** necessarily been approved by medical practioneers.

The reader should not use these remedies instead of, or in addition to, usual contempory medical procedures.

REMEDIES FOR:

Earache
Stomachache
Headache
Toothache

UPSET STOMACH

When my Grandpa Leland Rousman was growing up on a farm southwest of Morning Sun, he would occasionally get a stomachache. His stepmother, Mabel, had a remedy for stomachaches, no matter what the cause.

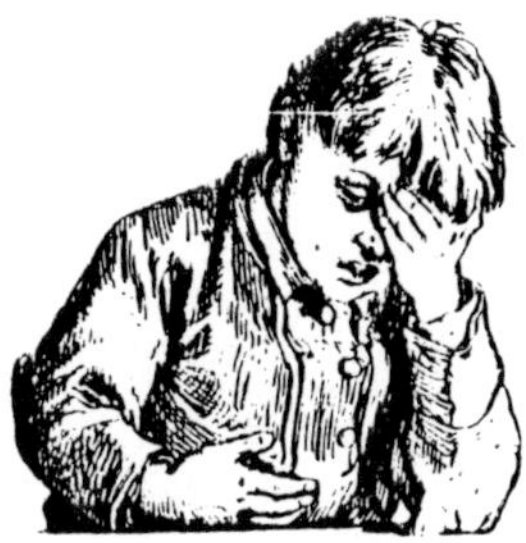

She would mix a very small amount of the spice ginger with a large glass of hot water, stirring until it dissolved. She would then have my grandpa drink that. She called it "Ginger Tea." He called it awful. If the stomachache persisted, she would mix up another glass of the "tea". Grandpa usually thought one glass was enough, but Mabel would always make two!

The stomachache would always subside. No one ever really knew if the stomachache just went away by itself or if the tea helped.

—by Crystal Housman

HEADACHES

Some old remedies seem unlikely to have helped the ailment, but most were applied at least near the area of pain or discomfort.

A popular one was putting a "cold cloth" on the forehead for a headache. When headaches bothered Midwest ladies, they would sit down, soak

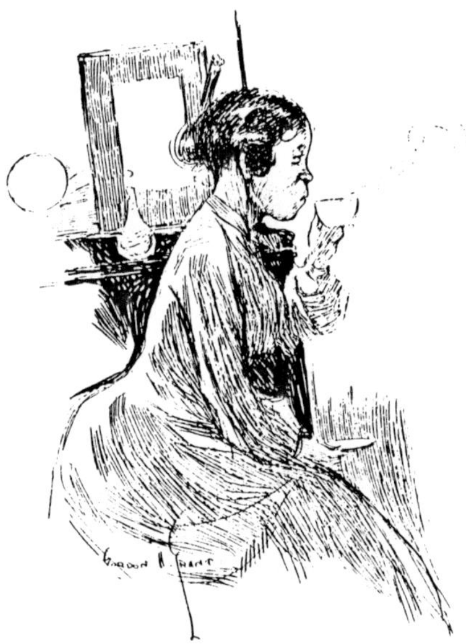

their feet in hot mustard water, lay a cold wet cloth on their stomaches, take two tablespoons of lemon juice, and wait for their headaches to go away.

—*By Seth Stone*

MINT TEA

Mint tea was used for an upset stomach of diarrhea. Mint plants grew easily in flower gardens. The plant looks like a weed, but isn't. When the leaf is broken off, it has a strong smell of mint. The mint leaves would be dried and preserved for winter use.

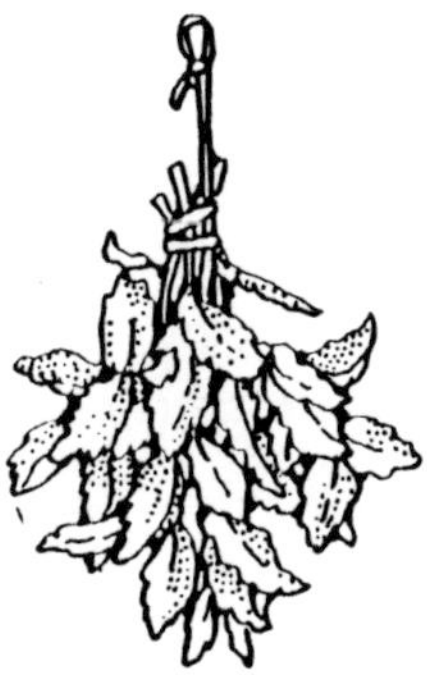

MINT

Mint tea would consist of crushed mint leaves with a little sugar. Water would be added and the leaves and water mixture would be boiled. The tea would be strain ed and diluted if too strong to use the way it came out of the pot.

Mint tea soothed the stomach. Today liquids are known to be the best thing for diarrhea, and warm weak tea is often the first thing a stomach will keep down.

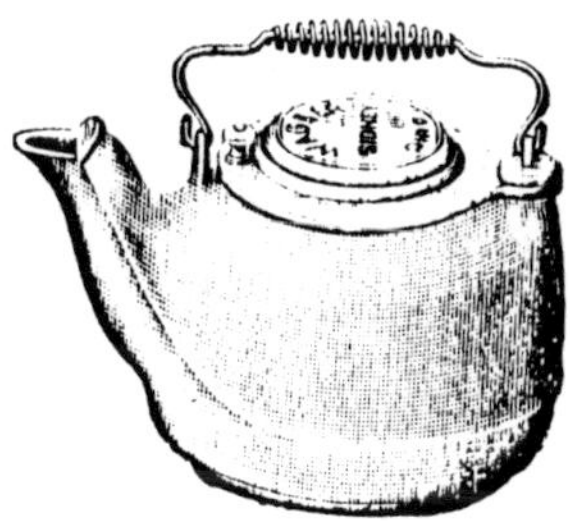

—by Lindsey Whipple

SMOKE, THE EARS' BEST FRIEND

In the days when there weren't antibiotics, infected ears were very painful. Most families were affected by an earache one time or another.

Ron Cross of Wapello tells of the time he had a horrible earache one summer day during the depression. His grandfather went into the woods and peeled off a fresh piece of bark from a birch tree. Then he rolled some fresh tobacco in the birch bark.

The old man then dipped the end of the homemade cigarette into some oil and lit it.

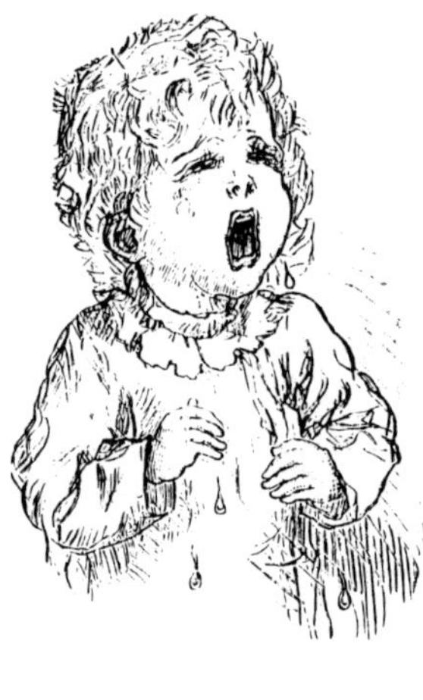

Once that cigarette was burning, he would blow smoke into Ron's ear, killing the infection.

—by Travis Lowe

CIGAR 'N ACHES

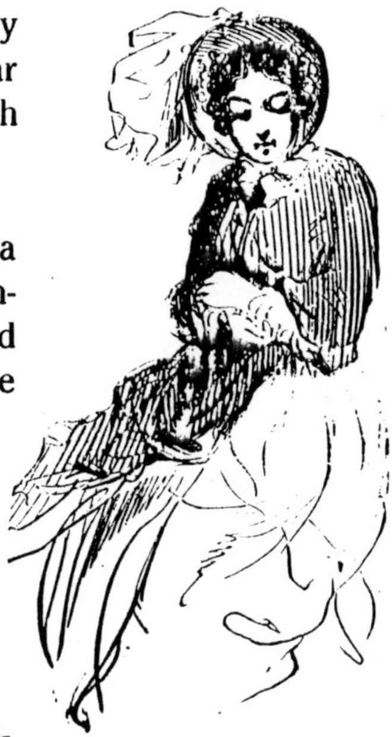

During the 1920s, Marion Langstaff, my grandmother, lived near Oakville on a farm with my grandfather.

One day my grandma had a terrible toothache. She had it so bad that she tried to pull the tooth out, but she couldn't.

Grandma walked to the store to get something for the pain, and while telling of her bad toothache, a man told her to try some cigar smoke. He said that cigar smoke would help toothaches.

So Marion bought one, lit it, and took a big mouthful of smoke. After about five seconds, she coughed the smoke out and found the tooth already hurting less.

Marion kept the cigar around just in case she ever needed it again.

—by Stephen Brown

SMOKE TO HELP EARACHES

When my cousins were little, my family would always go to Grandma and Grandpa Gersts' for Sunday afternoon and evening in Oakville.

My Dad and two of his brothers smoked. My cousins were always having earaches, and this one night one of them had one.

Poor Laura had a terrible earache and cried and cried and nothing would settle her down. Little Laura was only about four years old.

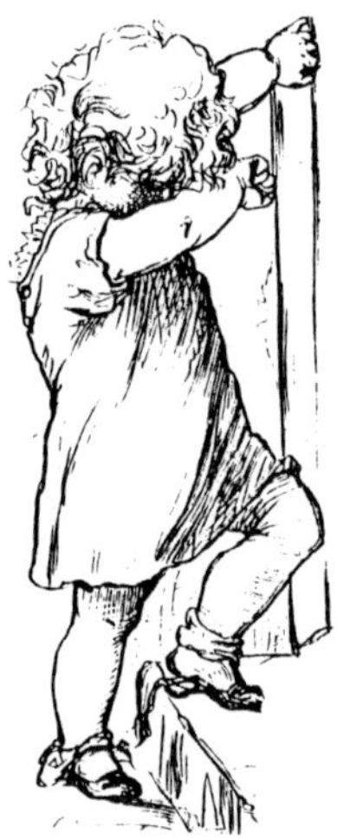

The grownups did everything to try to get that earache to stop, and finally someone came up with a new idea.

"Blow smoke in her ear, that will fix it."

So somebody did, they blew smoke right in her ear. He did this several times. In between times he blew smoke rings to make Laura feel good. For a while she tried to catch those smoke rings, but she soon dropped off to sleep, feeling real good.

—by Bobby Gerst

MY EAR HURTS

As a child, whenever my Grandma Whipple got an earache, she just had to suffer for a while. There was no money for doctors and medicine back then in our family.

"We only went to the doctor if our parents thought we might die!"

And, many children did die because good medicine was hard to get or expensive.

Great Grandma Rauhaus put sweet oil drops in little Virginia's ears. Sometimes they would take the hot

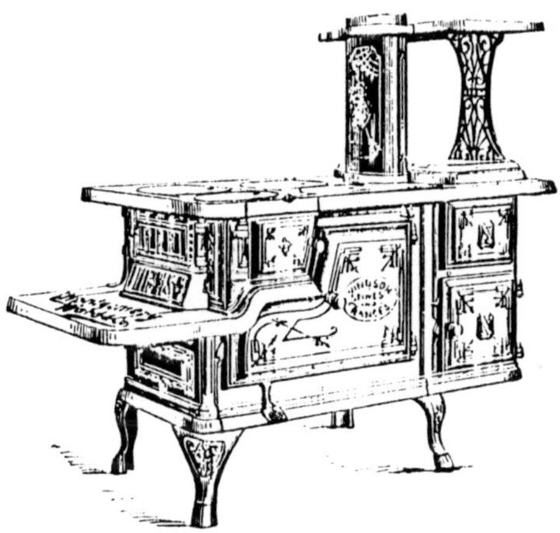

stove lids off and wrap them in newspaper, and use those to lay their heads on for the warmth to get relief.

by Lindsey WhippLe

HEATED SALT BAG

When my grandmother, Laurie Sherry Dorothy, was a little girl growing up in the 1930s near Davenport, many home medicine remedies were widely used, as money in those times was scarce.

One commonly used remedy for earaches was a heated salt bag. A scrap piece of clean cloth was wrapped around some table salt.

The salt was then heated on the stove, and held on the ear or put on a pillow.

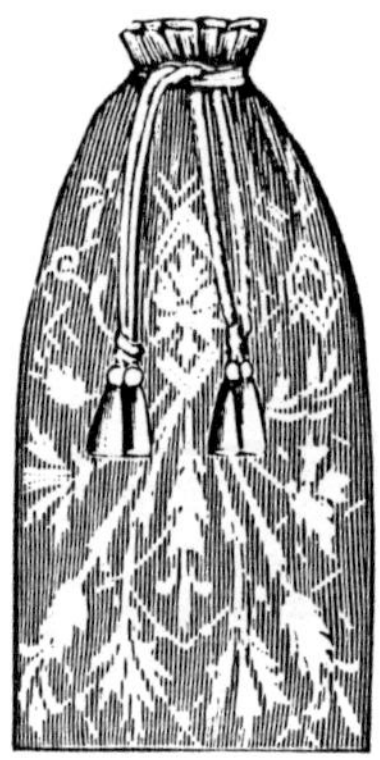

According to Grandma, the warm bag seemed to work real well in helping the pain of an earache.

—by Bob Hodges

A REMEDY FOR COLIC

When my Grandma Fletcher was a little girl back in the early 1920s, she lived near Columbus Junction. She remembers going out to pick peppermint for her mother.

The leaves were used as a home remedy for babies that were suffering from the colic or had bad tummyaches. Those leaves were steeped in hot water, just like you were making tea. the "tea" was then cooled to where the baby could drink it. A few drops of that was all that it took to relieve its tummyache.

My Grandma Fletcher remembers this remedy when she became a mother herself. She said that she made this "pepperment tea" for her first baby when it cried with the pains of colic.

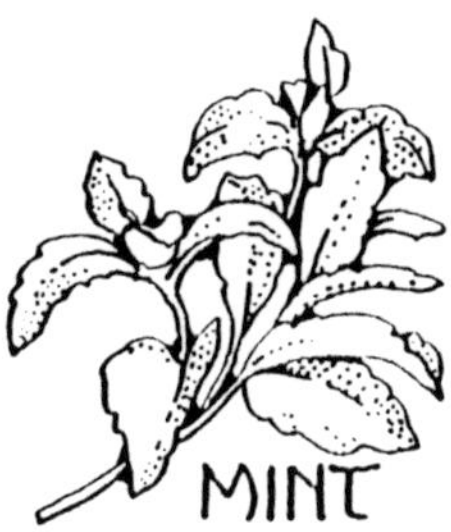

Grandma said she was never sure whether it was something in the peppermint leaves or just something warm in the baby's stomach that seemed to do the trick and ease the pain.

—by Daniel Bryant

UPSET STOMACHES

I found out from Vicky Housman in Fort Madison that when she was growing up and had a terrible stomachache, her parents would give her a full eight-ounce glass of warm water with about a teaspoon full of baking soda mixed in with it.

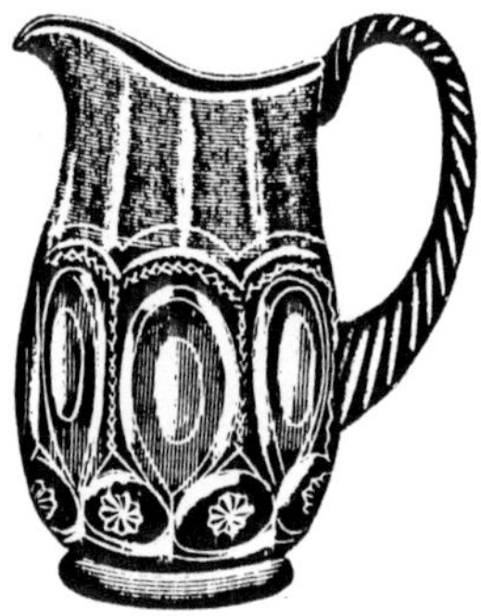

She had to drink this mixture and then go to bed and get a good night's sleep. During the night, the baking soda and water mixture was working to soothe her stomach, and it made her feel better.

If that stomachache wasn't gone when she got up in the morning she'd have to go through the whole thing again. Usually the second dose did the trick.

—by Crystal Housman

WARM MILK ON TOAST

Some thirty years ago in Van Buren County, my cousin, Jean McIntosh, remembers eating warm milk on toast as a remedy for an upset stomach.

Her grandmother, my great-grandmother, Mabel Dorothy, would prepare this remedy for her and the rest of the family.

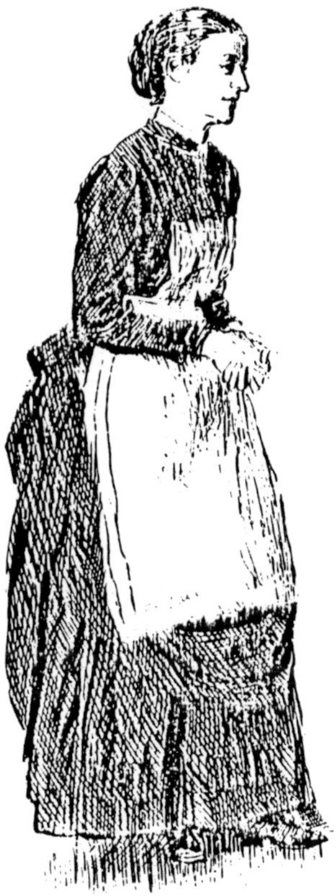

Mabel would make toast, heat some milk, and pour the warm milk over the toast in the bowl.

My grandfather, Jack Dorothy, of Keosauqua also remembers this remedy, and told me about it.

"Sometimes Mabel would put brown sugar on the toast to make it taste a little sweeter."

—by Bob Hodges

A COLICY BABY

When my sister was a little baby, she was very fussy. She was my Mom's first baby, and my Mom didn't want to let her cry. She took her to the doctor who said there was nothing wrong with the child and my mother should go ahead and let her cry.

My parents lived in a very small home in Iowa City. When my sister cried, she could be heard right through the walls on the outside.

One day, after trying everything, Mom laid my sister down in her crib where she could see her, and Mother started to clean the carpet.

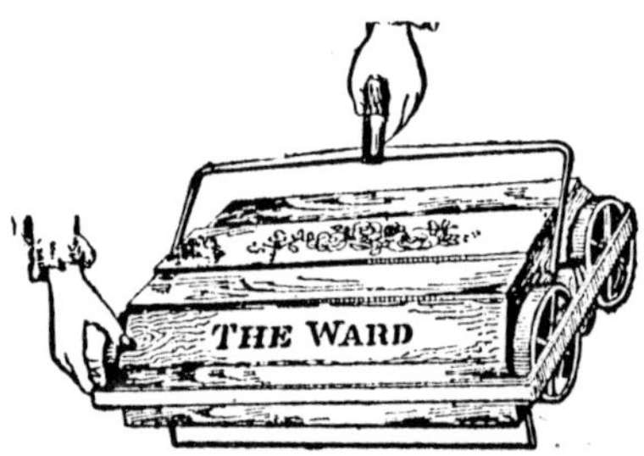

Mother glanced toward the crib to check on my sister. Much to her surprize, she was asleep. The next time she did that, it had the same result. The hum of that cleaner seemed to do the job.

—by Erin Armstrong

BAKING SODA AND TEETH

My Uncle Joe Langstaff lived in Louisa County many years ago.

Uncle Joe always took pride in this teeth, and tried to take good care of them. He was not fond of dentists. And he was definitely not fond of false teeth. He was determined to never let this teeth get so bad that they had to be pulled.

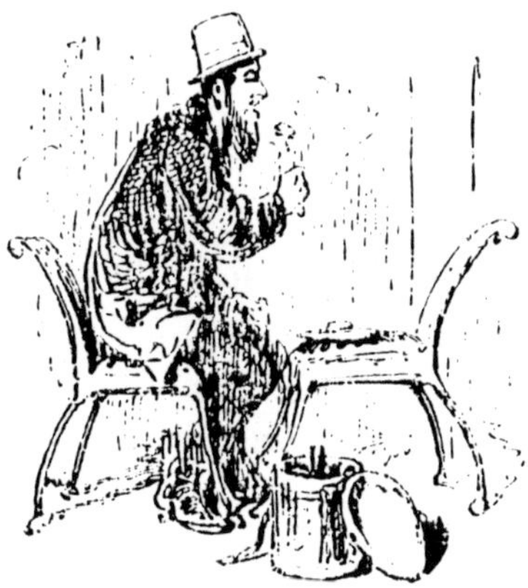

Joe brushed his teeth often, but when he would run out of toothpaste, he'd use baking soda. He said it tasted kind of gritty, but it did a good job of cleaning his teeth.

Either the toothpaste, or the baking soda, or Uncle Joe's persistence paid off. He didn't lose them.

—by Stephen Brown

OUT OF TOOTHPASTE

Growing up on a farm meant going to town was a whole-day event, and groceries were bought once month. There were times you learned to make do with what you had on hand. Some of those times, the substitute item turned out to be as good as the "store-bought" item.

One morning my mom's family found themselves without toothpaste. Now, Mom was used to putting toothpaste on her brush each time and just plain figured a person couldn't brush teeth if there wasn't any toothpaste.

Her mother insisted that she use just water.

"It will work fine and you might want to use a little soda to freshen your mouth a little more.

And, sure enough, it worked great. And just this year a dentist told me I could use just plain water if I was out of toothpaste.

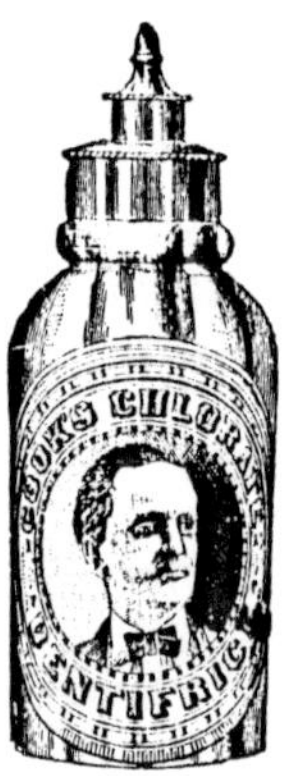

"Don't worry, it will work just fine."

I guess good advice stand-the test of time after all.

—by Erin Armstrong

ALKA SELZER AND VICK'S VAPORUB

Alka Selzer and Vick's Vaporub are products that remain on grocery and drugstore shelves today, but my father, Mike Hodges, remembers that his grandfather, Arthur Poling, had a different way of using these products.

My dad spent about one weekend a month with his grandparents while he was growing up.

They lived on a farm near Keosauqua in Van Buren County, where Great-Grandpa Poling still lives.

Alka Selzer was used not only for the usual upset stomach as prescribed, but also for almost any internal ailment.

Whatever the problem, the prescription was the same. Alka Selzer was used for inside problems and Vick's Vaporub for outside ones.

—by Bob Hodges

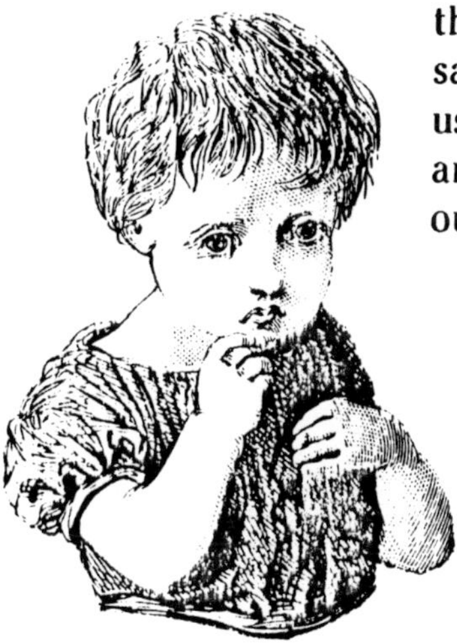

REMEDIES FOR:

Cuts
Wounds

SALT FOR BLEEDING

When Carol Rawhouser was a child, her family lived on a farm in southeast Iowa.

The Rawhouser family raised horses and had a special pasture for them. Unfortunately, there were some sharp hazards in that pasture, including a long nail that dug deep into the side of Honey, Carol's horse, when she fell on it.

The wound refused to stop bleeding. Sick with worry, Carol pushed some table salt into the cut and wrapped it as best she could. She knew Honey could die.

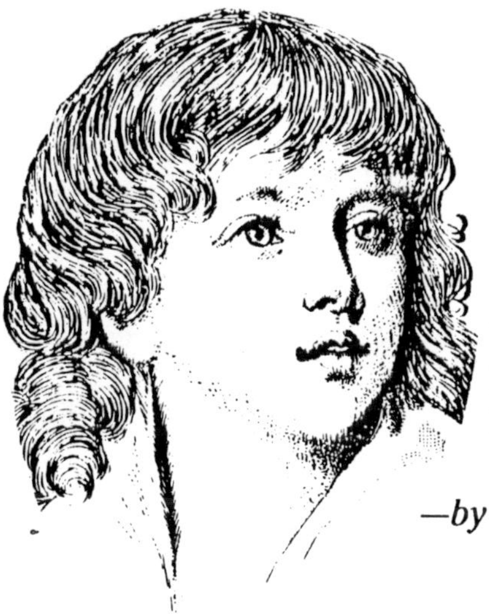

But the salt did the trick, and her beloved little mare recovered from her ordeal.

The cut didn't even leave a scar on Honey.

—by Les Hollingsworth

BAD CUT

When my Great Uncle John was a little boy back in the 1930s on a farm four miles southwest of Morning Sun, he used to play outside a lot. And, he'd get hurt, too.

One time when my uncle was outside playing, he was standing by his father watching him cut a tree down.

Now even knowing the boy was there, his father dropped his axe, and it landed right on Uncle John's foot. It made a nasty cut right on the top.

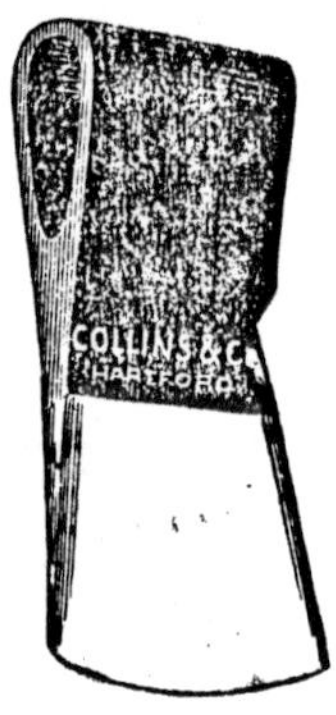

Uncle John's father rushed him to the house as quickly as he could.

Hurriedly they washed his foot off, but they couldn't get the bleeding to stop, even with a real tight bandage.

They were afraid to go to the doctor's since it was such a long trip, and they feared the boy would lose too much blood.

John's mother took a cobweb and mixed it with sugar and put that on the cut, then wrapped it well. By morning it was already starting to heal.

—by Crystal Housman

KEROSENE FOR CUTS

In the 1920s money was scarce and doctors were, too.

Once, Orville Schmeiser on a farm near Wapello was using a buck knife to carve a wooden recorder, which is a flute-like instrument. His knife slid across the stick into his arm, cutting into his muscle.

Blood spurted onto the ground as the screaming boy took off for the house.

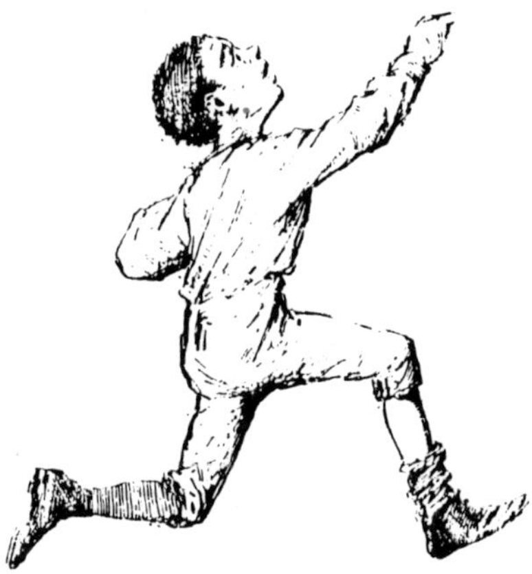

His mother immediately saw what had happened and grabbed a kerosene lamp from the table. She poured kerosene into that wound to stop the bleeding and to keep it from getting infected. It worked real well.

—by Aaron Locke

A WAR WOUND

My grandfather, Doug Langstaff, was in combat when he was a soldier in the army.

One time, during battle, he was shot in the shoulder and was bleeding badly.

No one seemed to know where a doctor or a medic was so his friends had to take care of him themselves.

One of the men suggested he put some chewing tobacco on the wound. Well, that didn't sound very sanitary, but they had to do something to stop the bleeding.

So one of the men put some chewing tobacco on the wound and it did stop the bleeding. The pain seemed to become much less severe then, too.

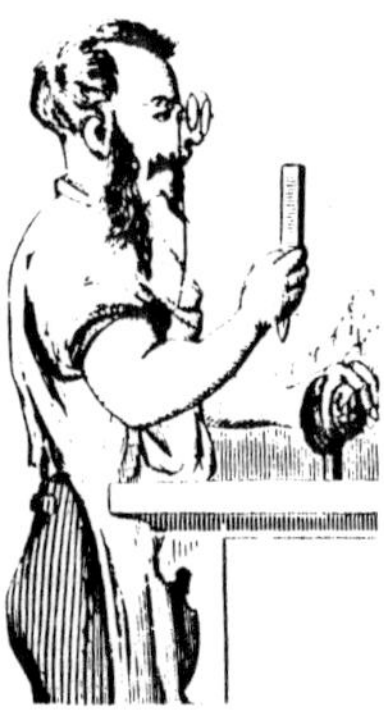

When the men finally got my grandfather to a doctor two days later, the man was amazed at the lack of infection in the wound.

But, it sure doesn't sound very sanitary to me.

—by Stephen Brown

POTATOES AND PUNCTURES

When Gary Samuels was growing up in the 1930s near Morning Sun, they had something to cure anything.

For puncture wounds, they had to do something to draw out the "poison," so they'd cut a potato

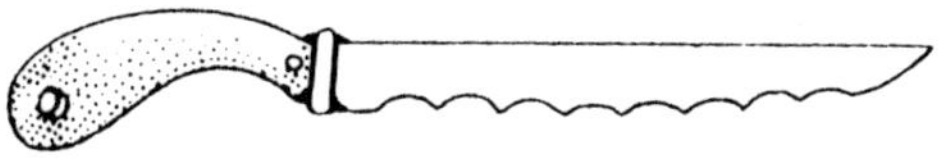

to just the right size to cover the wound and let it set there for a while. Then, they'd take it off and pitch the potato.

Sometimes they'd grate the potato and put a handful of the gratings on the wound. Then they would tie a clean rag over it. This seemed to work well for wounds that had already gotten infected.

We don't know why this seemed to work, but it did. Maybe there is something in potatoes we don't know about.

—by Tina Samuels

NO BANDAGES

"Edna, get that cloth of yours, will ya? I've got an oozing cut from a nail that I was hammering. My hand got in the way, and I hammered my hand instead of the nail."

"Hadley, you really should be more careful than you are."

"I know, I know. Just get me that cloth."

Edna got the cloth for him and started the remedy that she knew. She had to put it over the stove until it got brown. That kills the germs and makes it sterile.

Edna then let the cloth cool before putting it on the cut.

This old-fashioned remedy does a lot toward preventing infection.

Thus was the life of Edna and Hadley Heater during most of their married lives in Wapello where they farmed.

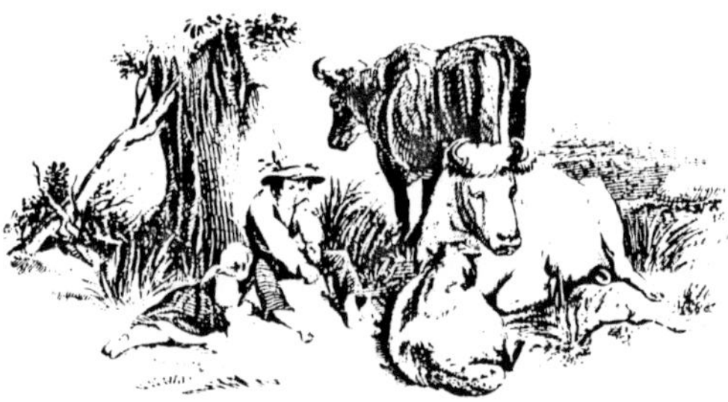

—by Jaime Heater

STOPPING BLEEDING CUTS

When Bub Krieger from Mt. Union got a cut on the farm, his parents didn't take him to the doctor. Doctors were scarce and they came only for emergencies. If there was a remedy, people would use it. Drugs weren't available very much. Home remedies were handed down within a family.

When Bub went howling to this mother, she would first wash the cut with homemade soap and some water. Then, she'd pour turpentine over the cut to try to keep down infection.

Bub says the soap stung simply awful, especially if his mother had to scrub some to get the dirt out. And then, he knew the mighty turpentine would be next. Oh, but that would sting!

If the cut kept bleeding, his mother would wrap it tightly with a rag to put pressure on it. This would help stop the bleeding.

Those rags Bud's mother used would first be heated over the stove to kill the germs.

Probably the hardest part of the whole thing was to get a young farm boy to lie still long enough to do all this.

—by Anna Reighard

TO STOP BLEEDING

Before antibiotics were really available, people had their own favorite remedies for treating minor wounds and sicknesses. Some of them seem kind of strange now, but the people who used them claimed they worked quite well.

Bob Beckett of Argyle, remembers what he used to use to stop bleeding when one of his family got cut. He would go to the barn and collect a handful of cobwebs. He would put sugar on the cobwebs and put them on the wound until the bleeding stopped.

Harrison and Katherine Pezley of rural Charleston had another method of stopping a wound from bleeding. They would mix flour and sugar together, and apply this to the cut.

Hugh and Lottie Vee Tweedy of rural Montrose would fight infection with turpentine. When one of their twelve children would step on a rusty nail or something else, they would have them soak the wound in turpentine.

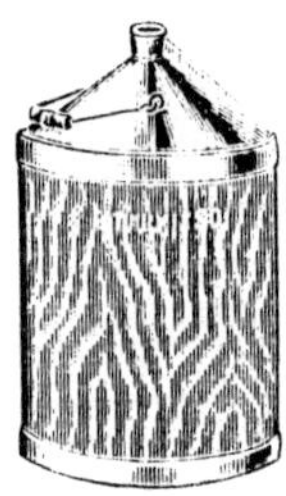

And the bare feet of twelve children must certainly have picked up a lot of nails through the years.

—by Nicole Simmons

REMEDIES FOR:

This 'n That

PREMATURE BIRTH

Mildred Simmons of Fort Madison tells of when her oldest sister was born to Alberta Ellen White.

Alberta was born prematurely and weighed only one and a half pounds. The doctor came to the house for the delivery, that being a common practice in those days around the turn of the century.

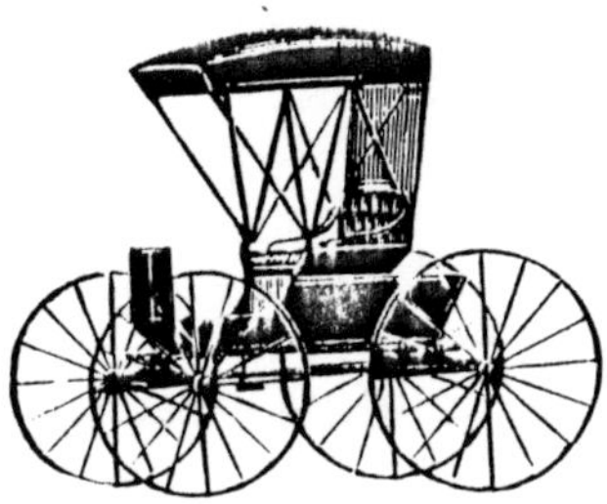

Since the doctor didn't have access to modern medical devices such as an incubator, he improvised.

Alberta was put in a cigar box and then in a warm oven as a makeshift incubator.

That new little baby was fed milk from an eyedropper until she was strong enough to nurse on her own.

It worked pretty well since Alberta is alive yet today and living in Florida.

—by Nichole Simmons

FLAX SEED

During the depression lots of people went blind because of inadequate medical care when they had gotten something in their eyes.

Ron Cross of Wapello remembers that when he had gotten something in his eye, his grandfather would find some flax seed.

Normally the seeds of flax are used to make linseed oil, but in this remedy they would find another use.

The little seed was very slick and would have the handy property of attracting an object in the eye right to itself. Yet, the flax seed was big enough that it wouldn't get lost in the eye, making its own problem.

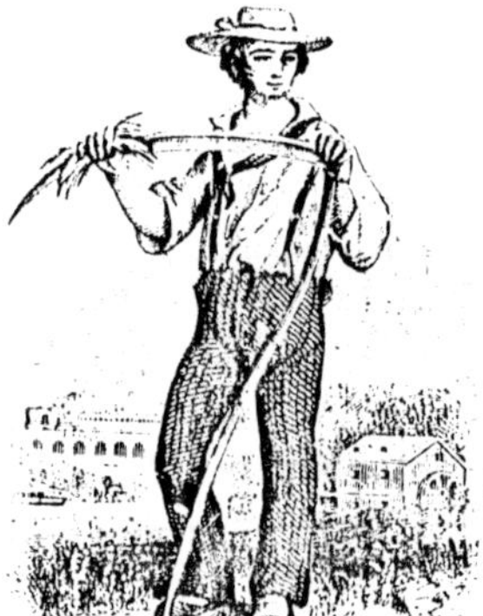

—*by Travis Lowe*

LEMON 'N SUNLIGHT

When my mother and her sister were in their teens, they decided that their hair was ugly colors, and they needed to do something about it. Their mother, Mrs. Yoder, told them an old remedy for hair color.

This involved apple cider, vinegar, and lemon juice.

If you used this for a month or two, it was supposed to make your hair lighter. But, it was also necessary that the girls go out in the sunlight, too.

After about two weeks, Gail thought Janell's hair was turning a green shade. Their brother said apples would start growing in their hair, but they kept rinsing and sunning. By the end of the summer, they were sure their hair was lighter, more luxurious, and nicer.

Looking back to that summer, the girls think how much trouble they went to. Today, something store-bought would do it a lot easier and faster.

—by Jaime Heater

TEAS

Here are some teas used years ago in Iowa:

Herb Teas

Dried sage or mint leaves, crush ¼ ounce.
Boil with ½ pint of water.
Steep and strain.
Cool, add sugar if desired.

Sage Tea

Make as above with ½ teaspoon of alum added.

Strawberry Leaf

Crush green leaves.
Apple on canker sores, or
Cook with water, strain and use as a mouth wash or gargle.

Blackberry Tea

The roots of blackberry or raspberry are boiled and strained . . . good for fevers and inflammations.

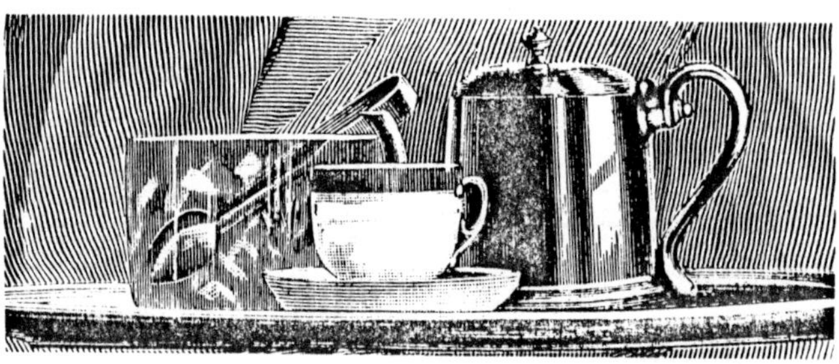

—by Lindsey Whipple

UNCONSTIPATING OIL AND SALT

In the depression years of the 1930s, jobs and money were scarce, and people relied on home remedies to cure injuries and illness.

Ron Cross remembers some of the old remedies.

Sometimes a bad stomachache was caused by constipation. A reliable laxative was Epsons Salts. Several teaspoons of it were stirred into a cup of water. The person drank the mixture, and usually within twenty-four hours he or she was unconstipated.

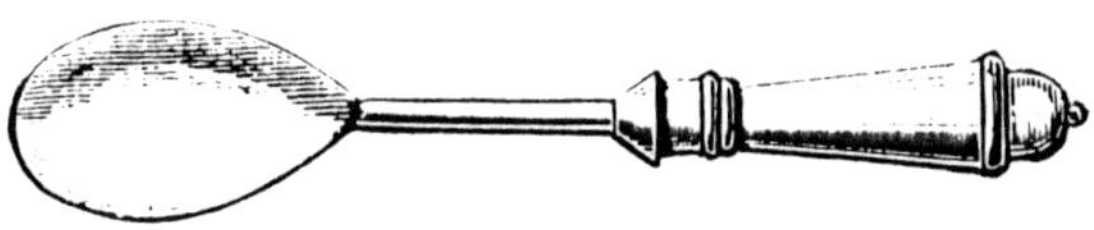

Another common laxative was caster oil. A tablespoon of castor oil was mixed into a glass of orange juice. One dose would usually take care of the problem, or at least make you wish you were cured.

—by Travis Lowe

DIAPER RASH

Ruth Yakle of Wapello tells about a remedy she used many years ago.

She would get a cup of flour and an iron skillet. She would put the skillet on the stove or over a candle and scorch the flour. Then, she'd let it cool and put in on cloth diapers. Doing this every day will cure a baby's rash.

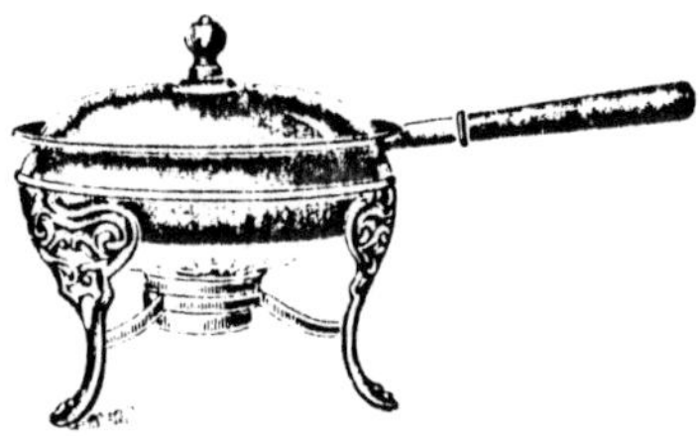

—by Travis Lowe

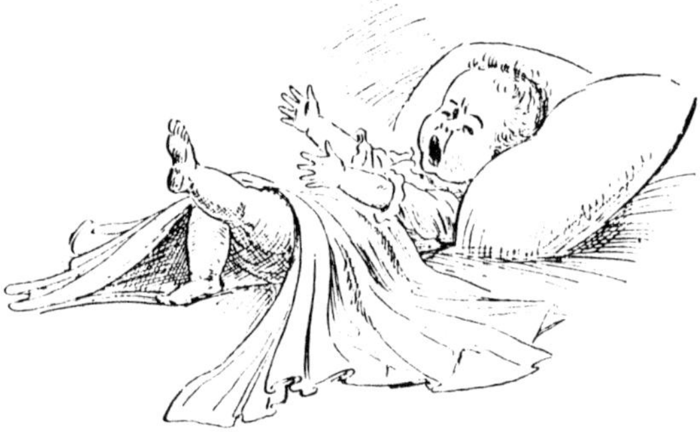

BACON FAT FOR BURNS

Shirley Foor used to use bacon fat or lard on a burn in Wapello.

She would take bacon fat and spread it on the burn and put a bandage on it. In a few weeks, the burn would be gone.

The way you get bacon fat is to save it from when you cook bacon. It is very easy to get that or lard from the meat that you cook.

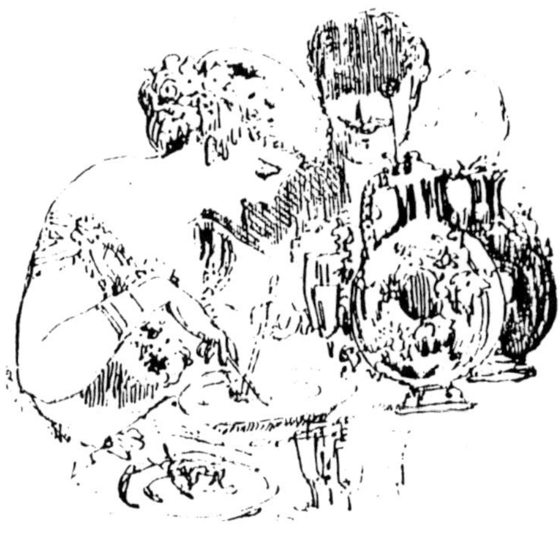

Bandaging the burn would protect it from germs and infection.

The fat prevents the bandage from sticking to the burned area.

—by Ryan Foor

BACON AS DRAWING SALVE

Peg is a lady that works with my mother, Barb Gerst, in a restaurant in Oakville.

Those ladies wash lots and lots of dishes so they have their hands in water very much. In the wintertime, their hands get so dry they get very badly chapped, even if they use hand lotion.

Sometimes Peg's fingers will crack right around the nails and get really sore.

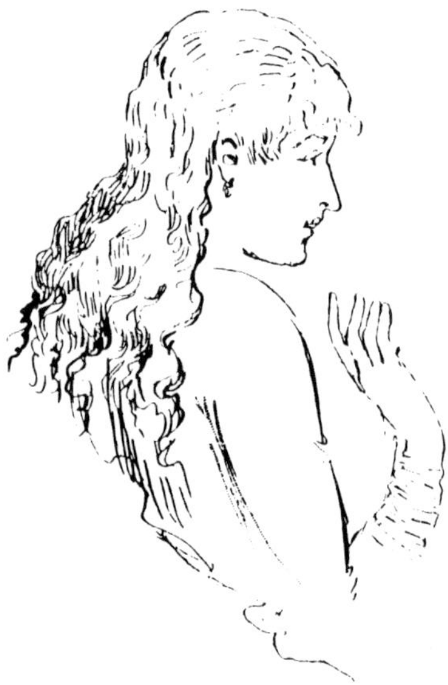

When this happens, she wraps a piece of bacon around the nail and leaves it overnight. It heals right up.

—by Bobby Gerst

REMEDIES FOR:

Bee Stings
Warts

BEE STINGS

Lois Bliven remembers so well that day in 1936 when she got stung by a bee while she was outside playing.

When she ran inside for help, her mother put a teaspoon or so of baking powder in a bowl and mixed enough water with it to make a paste.

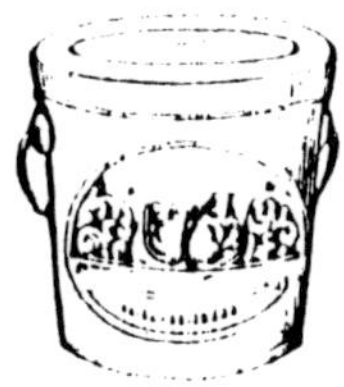

Quickly, she put that paste all over there on Lois's arm where that bee had gotten her.

She finished up by wrapping a bandage all around the arm.

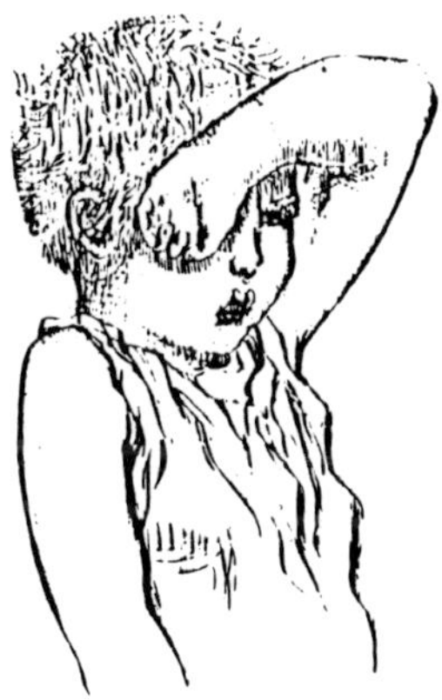

By morning that sting was cured and almost invisible.

—by Erin Spitznogle

BEE STINGS

When my Grandma Bonnie Dotson lived in Louisa County as a small child in the 1920s, she did something pretty silly. She sat on a bee's nest.

Can you imagine how much that must have hurt? She got lots and lots of bee stings on her bottom. So her mother, Pauline Eubanks put mud on the

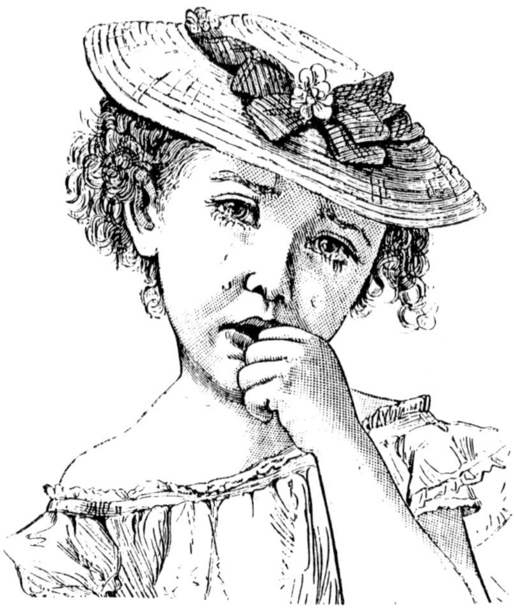

stings. She put lots of that wet, slimy mud on them. The stings were still there, but the mud took the hurt right out of them.

—by Jason Cross

GETTIN RID OF WARTS

One day Donna Yoder discovered a large wart on her forehead. She was afraid that burning the wart would hurt or leave a scar. Then she remembered an old remedy that her mother had used.

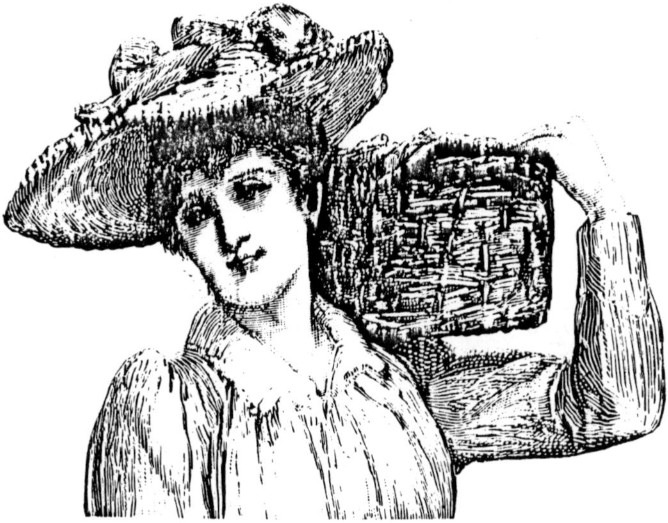

Donna cut off a slice of raw potato. It had to be nice and juicy, or it wouldn't work.

Every day for a month she rubbed the potato slice on her wart or taped a piece on there for fifteen or twenty minutes.

As the month passed, the wart got smaller and smaller; then it was gone.

—by Jaime Heater

CHICKEN BLOOD?

Everyone was giving my aunt, Carlyne Burge of Morning Sun, lots of advice on how to get rid of a wart. It was on her big toe and gave her lots of pain when she walked.

It hurt so much that she finally agreed to even try chicken blood, a remedy she got from Dollie Frank, a friend and neighbor.

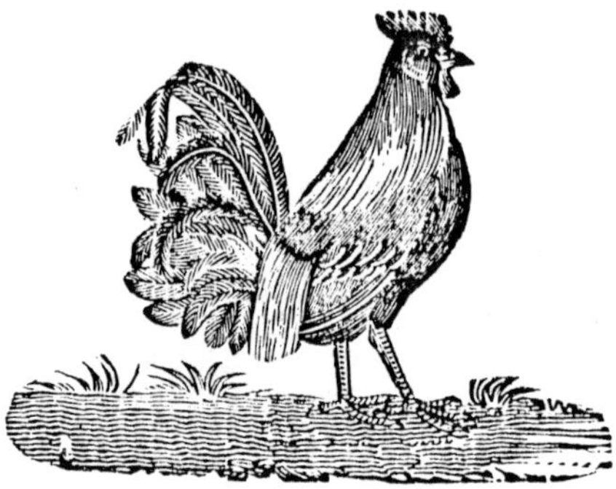

Fortunately it just happened to be chicken cleaning time, so Grandpa Glen Samuels cut off a chicken's head and put the blood on Carlyne's toe.

Carlyne figured it would be just awful, and it was.

Grandpa told her not to wash it off at all. Carlyne could hardly stand it, knowing that yucky blood was on her toe, but she minded. She wanted that wart gone.

Grandpa put more blood on that wart every day, and in a week it was gone.

—by Tina Samuels

MISSISSIPPI MUD FOR BEE STINGS

Years ago in Morning Sun, my grandma's friend, Barb Sands, was over for a visit.

The two of them were walking around in the garden when Barb got stung by a bee.

She started to cry because it really hurt. My grandma quickly picked up some dirt, spit on it just enough to make it sticky, and slapped that right on Barb's sting.

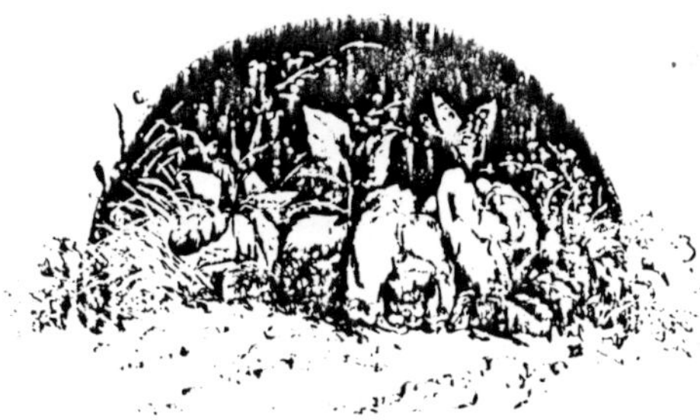

Barb was shocked to find that that sting felt a lot better right away.

I asked my grandma if that was some kind of special mud.

"Oh, no, jus' Mississippi River mud."

—by Jarett Ball

RUBS

Ointments were often used for various kinds of pain and for cuts, scrapes, and bruises. To get relief from stiff joints, boil equal parts of the bark of white

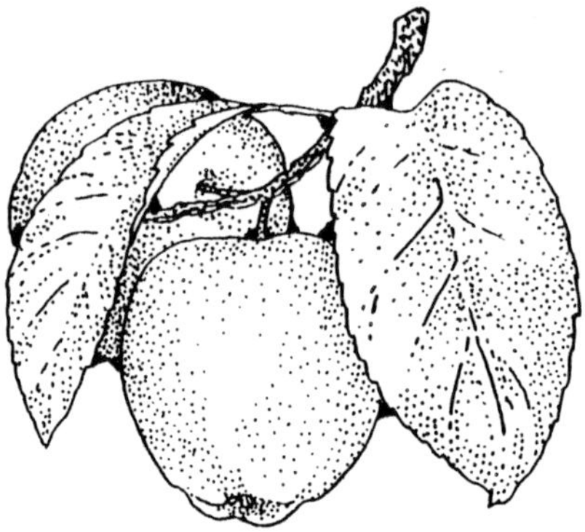

oak and sweet apple. Boil to a thick mixture, add an equal amount of goose grease, simmer, and let cool. Rub on sore and stiff joints as needed.

A handy ointment for cuts and scratches was made, years ago, from two ounces of beeswax, four ounces of resin, and six ounces of lard.

Melt all this together and cool. Add to the cooled mixture, four teaspoons of turpentine. You should do that outside to keep from burning the house down. It's excellent for preventing and curing infections.

—by Seth Stone

REMEDIES FOR:

Itches
Rashes

GALLING

If you've never been galled, you're lucky. It is a condition of your skin that is like an abrasion due to perspiration and the rubbing of clothes, especially in hot weather.

Duane Gerst from Oakville really got galled badly back when he was about ten years old.

Duane had been working in the field helping his father do some haying. He wore a shirt that seemed to be particularly abrasive and he sweat a lot.

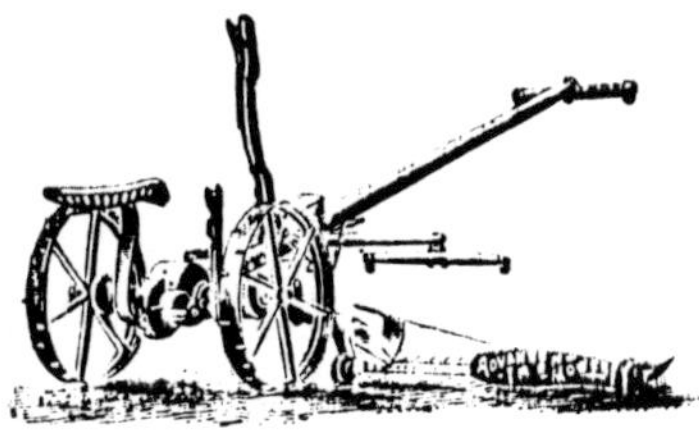

The underside of his arms became extremely raw and painful.

Duane suffered with that until someone told him about carrying a chunk of alum in his pocket. He didn't know how it worked, but it did. As soon as he did that, the galling cleared up.

—by Bobby Gerst

RELIEF FROM POISON IVY

My Grandpa Fletcher told about when he was a young man in the 1920s and had a real bad case of poison ivy on his arms.

That didn't slow down the need to keep working, though, and he was at the local blacksmith's with some parts from a plow to be repaired.

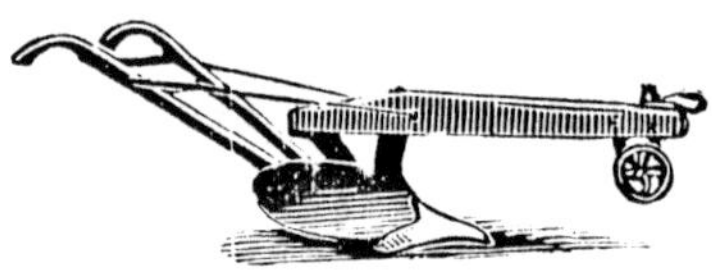

The blacksmith's shop was in the little village of Columbus Junction near the Iowa River.

While Grandpa was waiting, the blacksmith noticed Grandpa's arms, and asked if they bothered him.

When Grandpa confessed that they did, the man suggested that Grandpa wash his arms in the water the man had there in a wooden barrel.

Grandpa said that as soon as his arms hit that water and the smithy dunked his hot iron in, those arms felt much much better. He thought maybe it had to do with the iron scale in that water.

—by Daniel Bryant

PLANTIN

One good remedy for poison ivy grows right in most of our front yards. It is a plant called PLANTIN.

Barb Gerst had a lady tell her about this remedy while she was at a Farm Bureau Women's picnic. She said that all you have to do is to take a leaf and rub it between your fingers until it gets moist. then you rub the leaf over the poison ivy afflication.

If the poisoning is especially bad, this might hurt a little bit, but not a whole lot.

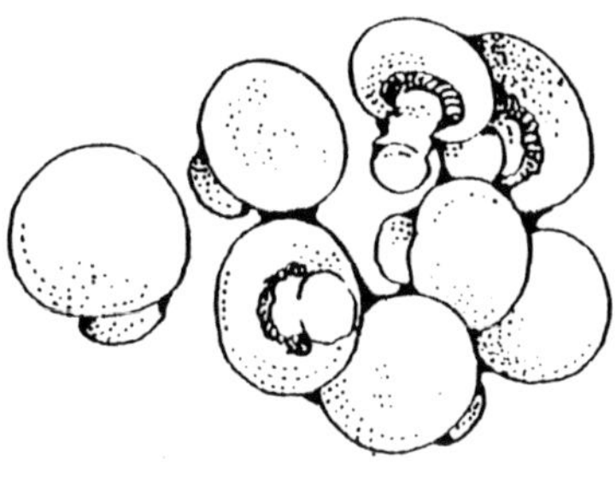

Barb had used this remedy several times because she likes to go mushroom hunting, and often ends up with a case of poison ivy from those mushroom excursions.

—by Bobby Gerst

THE ITCHY ITCH

Sometimes at my school, the kids get an itchy rash called scabies. It is caused by some tiny, tiny lice that you can't even see because they are so small.

Doctors prescribe a lotion that will kill the lice and stop the terrible itch.

When my Grandma Pogie was a little girl, growing up in Wapello, stopping that awful itch wasn't so easy. Woe unto the child who was caught itching by their mother! My grandma says her mother would rub her skin raw with lye soap. Great Grandma Dorthy Grimm would scrub and scrub until my Grandma Pogie was screaming for her to stop!

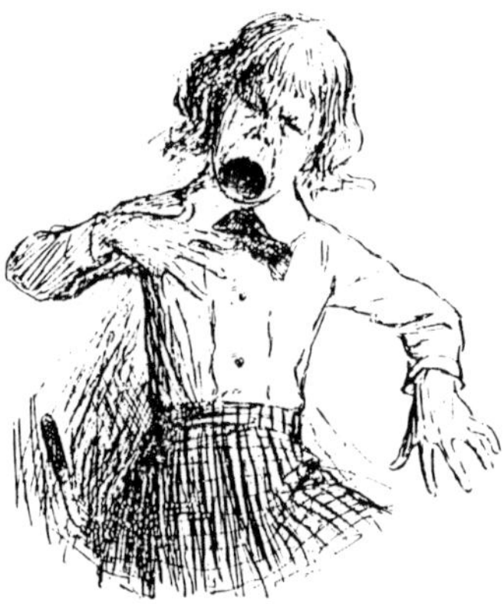

That might go on every day for several days until Great-Grandma Dorthy was sure she had killed every one of those little critters.

I'm glad we don't use lye soap anymore!

—by Lindsey Whipple

MEASLES

In my corner of Iowa, when a kid got the measle's years ago they would keep him in a darkened room.

One hot summer day when Joyce Mathes was a girl, she got that dreaded disease.

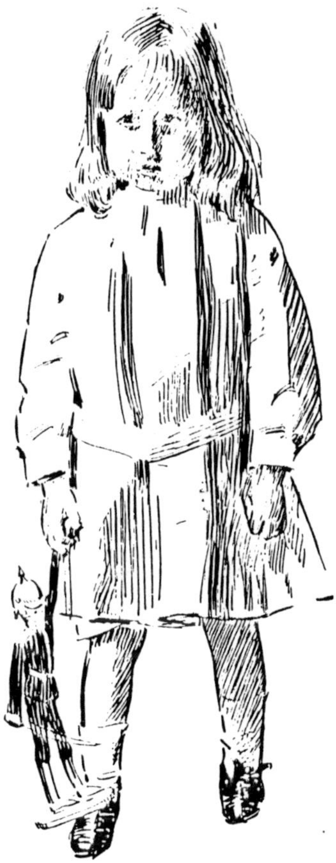

Grandma Bonnie Dotson put Joyce in a dark room. She belived that sunlight was supposed to hurt your eyes when you had the measles. Mrs. Dotson sure didn't want to risk the chance of Joyce losing her eyesight.

The measles' victims not only had to spend all that time in a dreary dark room, but they couldn't even read or other wise strain their eyes.

—by Jason Cross

CHILL BLAINE

In the early 1900s when Hugh and Lottie Vee Tweedy were raising their twelve children, they relied quite a bit on home remedies. Living on a farm some distance from town made going to town for medicines really difficult. Folks learned to use things they had around the house to treat medical problems.

When someone in the Tweedy family would get chill blaine, they would make a lotion from heavy cream to treat the problem.

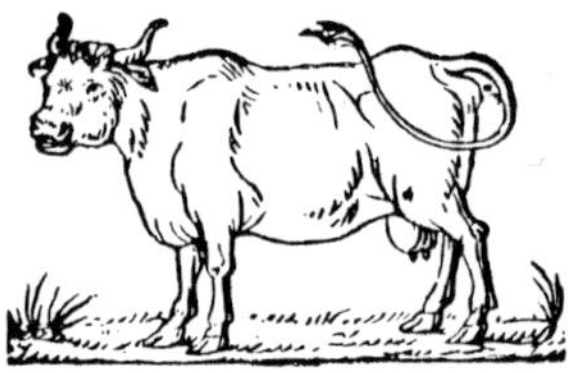

Chill blaine is itchy feet that is caused by the feet being cold for a long period of time. The old houses were not heated as nicely as ours are now, and the floors were usually cold in the winter.

Lottie would skim the heavy cream from the milk after they milked the cows and heat it on the back of the stove until it was very thick. That thick lotion was then rubbed on the feet at bedtime to help relieve the itching.

Actually, neither my teacher nor I have ever heard of chill blaine before.

—by Nicole Simmons

OATMEAL AND POX

The following is a natural remedy used on Matt Hagele of Wapello to relieve his itch due to chicken pox. Some doctors still prescribe this.

Cook a serving of oatmeal and put it in the center of a large square cloth, 15 to 18 inches on a side, draw up the corners, and tie them with a string to make a pouch.

Float this pouch in a tub of warm water, swishing it around until the water becomes silky, being careful not to break the bag. If you do, you have a terrible slimy mess.

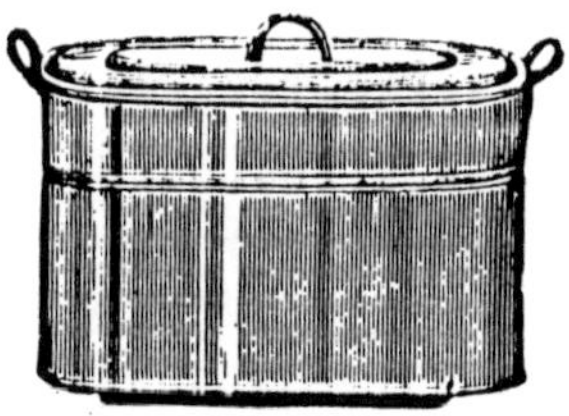

Let your child splash and play in this water . . . the pouch of oatmeal still in the tub. Be sure the water goes over all the scabs.

At first, do this two or three times day, depending on the itchiness of the scabs. As they get better, once a day is enough.

—by Mike Hagele

FLAKES ON YOUR SHOULDER

Even when my Grandma Pogie was a little girl, people worried about dry itchy scalp.

Folks coudn't go to the store and buy a store-bought lotion, so they used a home remedy. Here is one solution my Grandma used:

> "Wash the head every two days with a strong solution of salt water. Where salt water is not available, use a small hand-

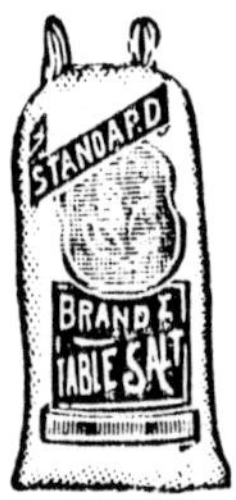

> ful of table salt mixed in a basin of water. Dip head in water, rub like the solution is a shampoo. Try not to get on skin, for it has a drying effect.

This has been known to remove dandruff where every other means has failed.

—by Allison Whipple

REMEDIES FOR:

Sore Throat
Croup

THE COMMON COLD

The search for the cure for the common cold has been going on for many years. In the early days here in Iowa, people caught cold and were miserable with coughs, sore throats, and headaches. The made up lots of remedies that were guaranteed to make them feel better.

One remedy for a bad cough called for soaking rock candy in whiskey and giving it to the person to suck on. Another popular cough rememdy suggested was a syrup made by combining one tablespoon of Vodka, one tablespoon of honey, and one tablespoon of lemon juice.

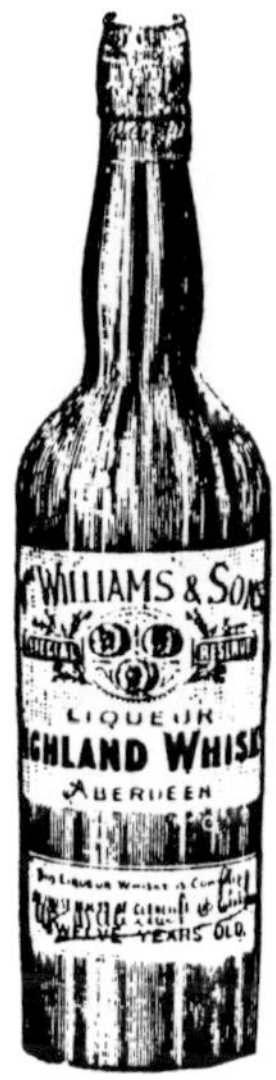

For children and others who preferred a soothing drink to a syrup for a cough, a "tea" could easily be made by boiling beef suet in milk and drinking it. Many mothers kept a cough remedy on hand by slicing up onions, covering them with sugar, and giving their children the juice as needed.

When Jane Jones of Clinton was a child in the early part of this century, her father, Clyde Bowers, a druggist, had many remedies that could be made with ingredients found in his drugstore. One of his favorites was concocted in the kitchen of their home.

To aid his daughters' recovery from colds, he would coarsely chop onions, boil them, stuff them

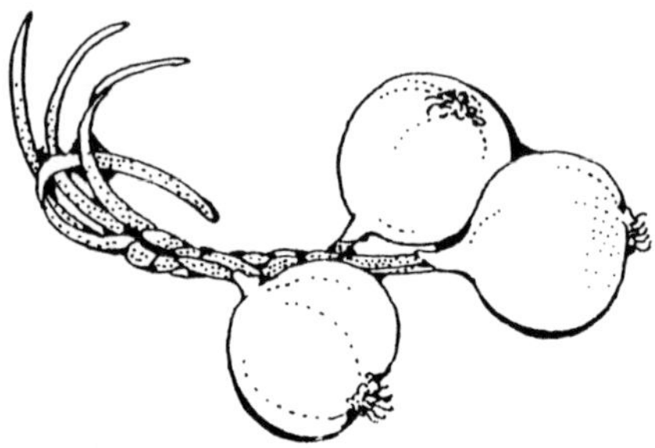

in an old long cotton sock and tie it closed. He would then warm up some bacon grease in a skillet, and roll the stocking stuffed with onions around in the grease until it was warm. This bag of onions was then put around the girls' necks and worn while sleeping.

Another of his remedies is still being used by his great-grandchildren. Many times, even prescription cough syrups cannot stop a childs cough in the night. When this happens, soak a washcloth in cold water, squeeze it out, fold it lengthwise into fourths, and place it around the child's neck. It will almost meet in the back. Be sure the front of the throat is covered. then fold a hand towel lengthwise and put it over the washcloth. Use large safety pins to fasten it in back. This resembles the soft neck braces worn for injuries today, but it is very comforting to children and very effective for children and adults.

by Seth Stone

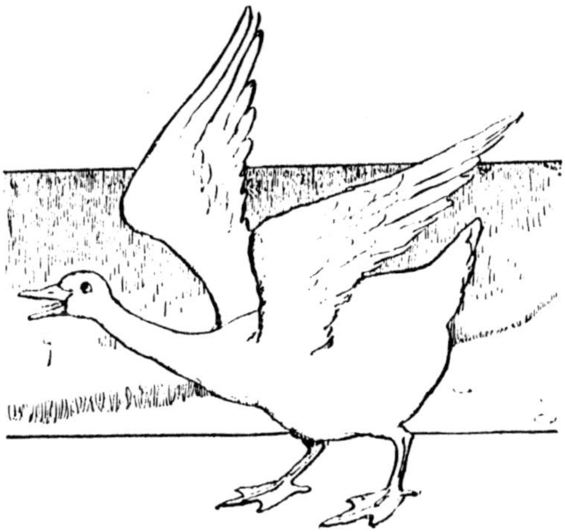

Lola Murry, an eighty-four-year-old great-grandmother of twelve, remembers when her chest congestion was treated by rubbing her chest with goose grease, and then covered it with a flannel cloth warmed in the cookstove.

by Seth Stone

TURPENTINE FOR CROUP

Croup has always been a problem with colds. It usually comes right on the heels of a cold. The larynx seems to swell and cause a rasping cough and difficulty in breating.

Humidifiers and hot steam from bathroom showers are often used now to provide relief from croup, but an old remedy is remembered by Louis Watson from near Morning Sun. This was to make a syrup.

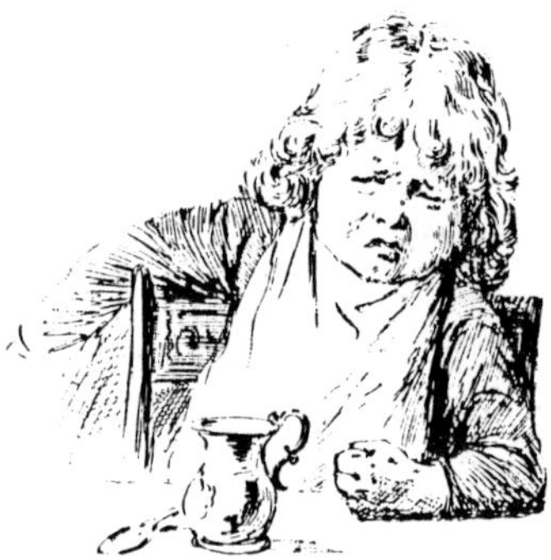

Melt a half cup of butter in a pan, and then put a small drop of turpentine in the butter. The mixture was taken as hot as possible and was often repeated every hour until the child felt some relief.

—by Jarett Ball

SUGAR AND ONIONS

One day in a small town near Davenport, in the early 1900s, Valeda Newman got an extremely bad case of the croup.

Valeda could hardly breathe and her attempts to do so were very painful. Ivan, her husband, compared her to the sound of a horse when she took a breath. Then she remembered . . . .

Her mother had a remedy that she had used. First Valeda cooked a cup of sugar and a cup of chopped onions together.

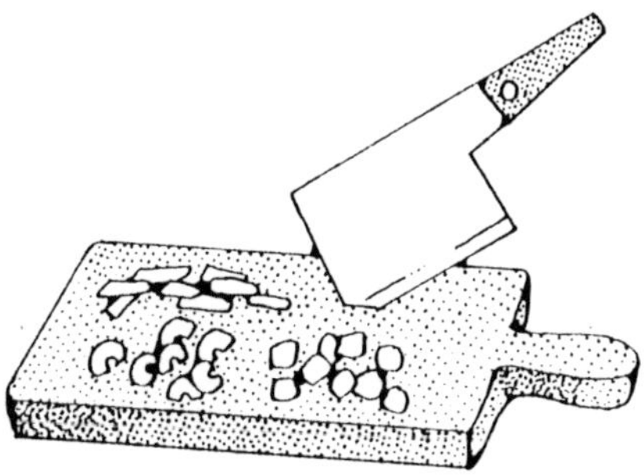

She cooked this in a pan until it turned to a liquid. She then took a spoonful of that every day for four days. Each time she had to just sip the medicine so it would go down her painful throat.

It worked for Valeda, but I think I'm glad I don't have to do it. I hate onions!

—*by Nathan Newman*

BLACK STRAP AND BAKING SODA

From down around Mediapolis comes another home remedy for the croup.

Many young children, when they caught a cold in the winter, would soon come down with that croup. If left untreated the mothers knew every breath would become a struggle.

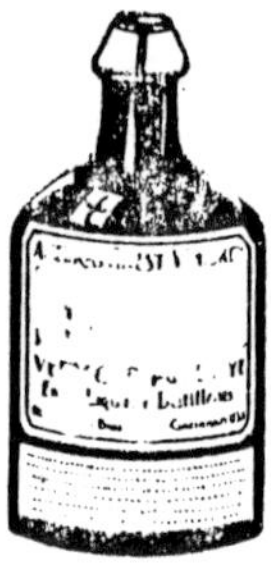

A time-tested treatment would be a homemade remedy of Black Strap molasses and baking soda.

First, about one third of a cup of that good old Black Strap molasses would be put into a pan.

Then a teaspoon of baking soda would be added. The baking soda would make the molasses foam up. After stirring, the prescription would be spoon-fed to the croupy youngster.

—by Denise Lanz

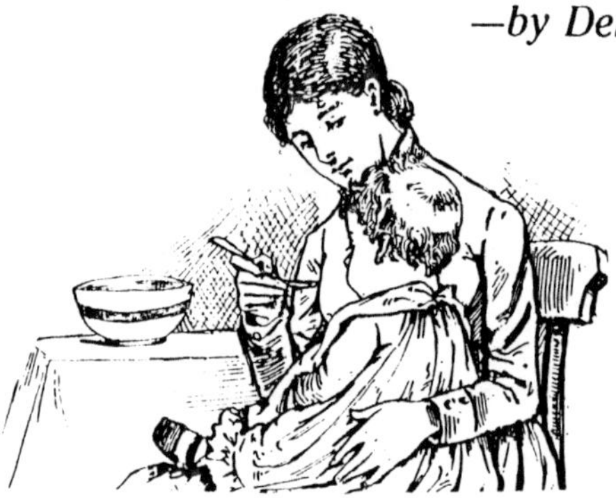

A CROUPY COUGH IN THE 1920s

Keith Larson, who grew up in Illinois City in the 1920s, remembers that his aunt, Miss Rachel Larson, would come into his room when he was a child, holding a kerosene lamp in one hand and a spoonful of sugar in the other, in which she had dropped a big drop of kerosene.

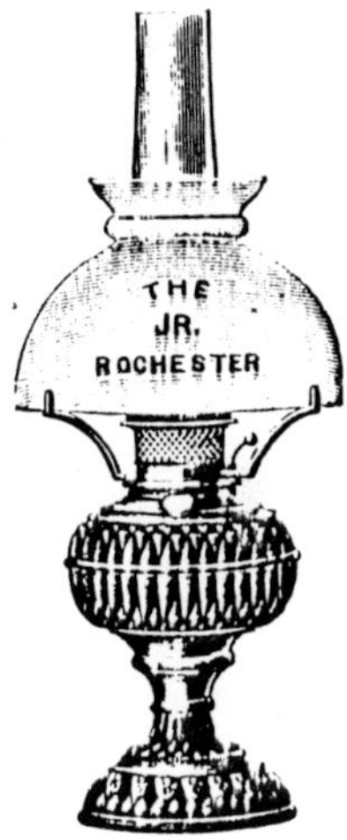

Keith knew full well that if the folks downstairs heard him cough in the night, they would be up with that sugar and kerosene concoction.

Try as he might, though, they would hear and Aunt Miss Rachel would come up and force that foul mixture down his unwilling throat.

Today we hurry to the drugstore for a cough remedy or even call the doctor. A vaporizer is a very commonly used item in our times for people to get some relief from a croupy cough.

But in the 1920s, if a home remedy could possibly be used instead of paying out money for medicine or a doctor, it was.

It is interesting to speculate as to how the sugar

and kerosene helped. Maybe it stimulated the salivary glands to help lubricate the throat.

We don't know how it worked, but lots of people thought it did.

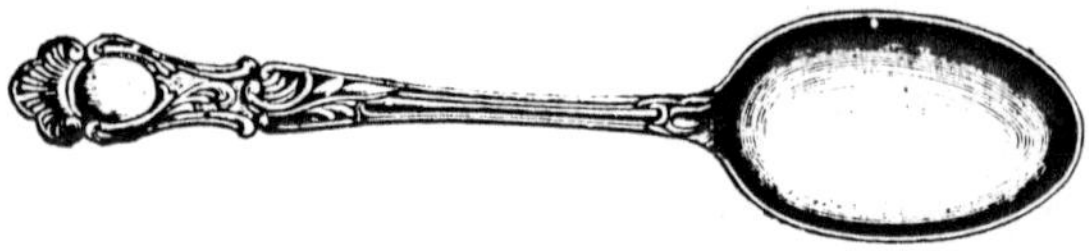

—by Anna Young

CROUP

When Virginia Tweety Pezley was growing up on a farm in rural Montrose, going to the doctor was done only when one was seriously sick or injured. The doctor was twenty miles away and the roads were bad, so gettin' there was slow going.

And with eleven brothers and sisters in the family, there wasn't what you'd call a lot of money left over for doctors. So, as true of most parents of the time, Hugh and Lottie Tweedy had their own methods for treating common illnesses.

The Tweedy family got many of their home remedy makins' right out of their own garden and from their own butchering of critters there on their place.

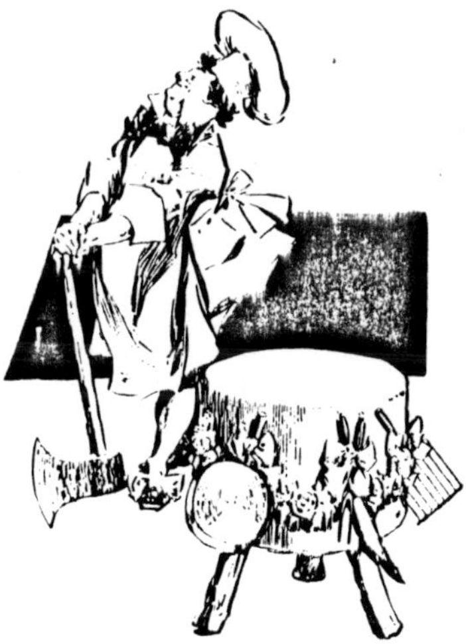

When one of the family would get the croup, a deep hacking cough, Lottie would mash up some of their onions and mix that with lard, the onions from their garden, and the lard from their hogs.

The mixture of onion and lard was then rubbed on the throat and chest of the sick child to stop the coughing.

One wonders which was the most effective, the rubbing of the mixture or the smelling of it.

—by Nicole Simmons

HOW TO GET RID OF A SORE THROAT

When my Grandma Fletcher was about twelve years old, she had a terrible sore throat. It was in the mid 1920s, and you didn't go to the doctor back then unless it was absolutely necessary.

Her father told her that he could cure that awful sore throat without a doctor.

So, he filled a teaspoon with sugar, then carefully poured a little whiskey out into that spoon.

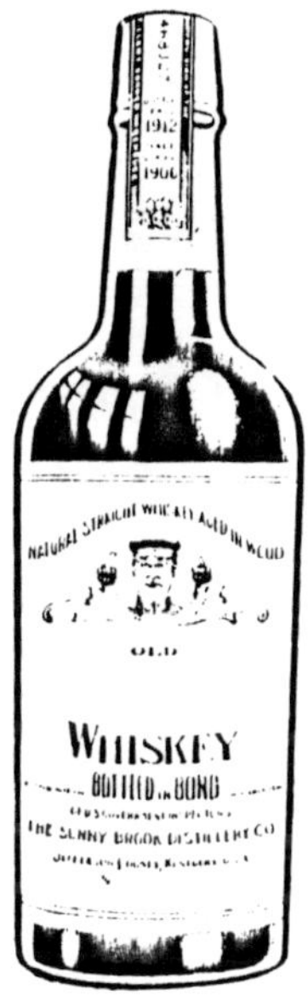

Grandma's father told her to sip the mixture slowly, swallowing just a little bit at a time.

The sugar made the whiskey stick to the throat, but it didn't help the taste any. Grandma said it really tasted bad, and it burned worse going down.

She couldn't remember if it helped her throat or if she just said it did to keep from getting a second dose of that awful stuff.

—by Dan Byrant

HOT LEMONADE

When my mother was growing up, they didn't go to doctors. My grandma used whatever they had to doctor the children.

In the wintertime, my mother would get some sore throats or a chest cold and out would come the Vick's jar and the lemons to make lemonade.

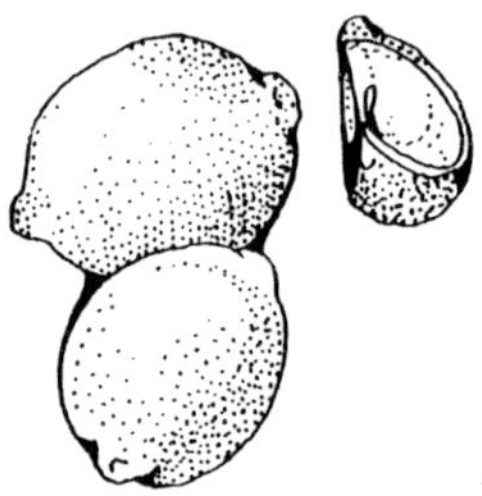

Grandma would heat some water up, squeeze a lemon into a cup of that hot water, and then add a tablespoon of honey.

She'd get that all stirred up and then make the kid drink it while it was still good and hot. That drink always seemed to vary between either real good, or just plain awful.

Meanwhile she would have the Vick's jar settin' on the stove so it would get good and warm and melted. Grandma would then rub that on my mother's chest and back and finally put a warm flannel rag around her neck.

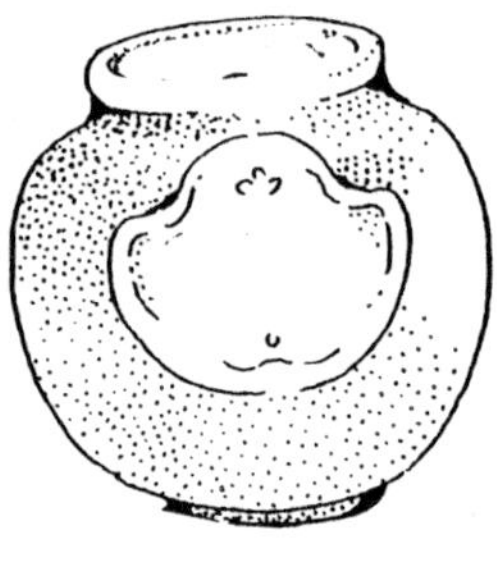

The lemonade would sooth the sore throat and help quiet the cough. Meanwhile the Vick's would break up the congestion in the chest.

Mother still likes to drink hot lemonade yet today when she has a sore throat.

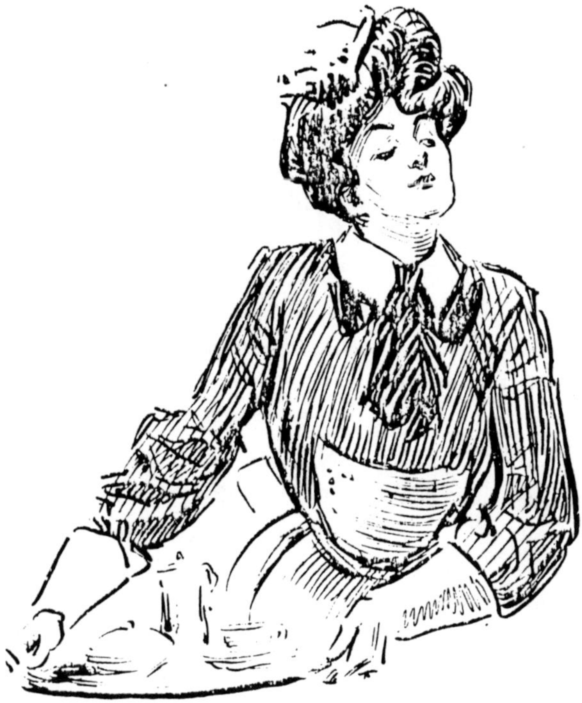

—by Bobby Gerst

COLDS AND SORE THROATS

I was talking to Loren and Mildred Simmons of Fort Madison about remedies they remembered that their parents used.

Loren recalled that when he would get a sore throat his parents, Macturion and Hazel Simmons of Fort Madison would put a generous amount of pepper on a piece of bacon rind.

Mrs. Simmons would put this against the side of the sore throat, pepper side in. She'd tie a rag around the whole thing to hold it on there.

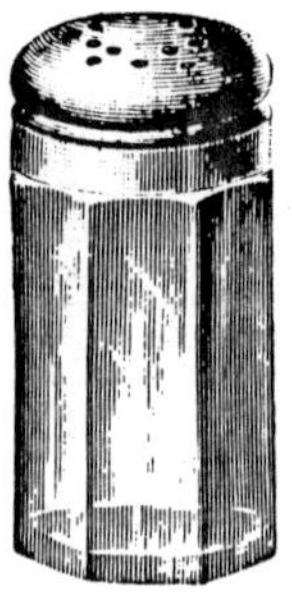

Mildred recalled that her mother, Ellen White in Fort Madison, would give her dad a cut-up onion in a cup of water.

This onion tea was supposed to be good for lots of things.

—by Nicole Simmons

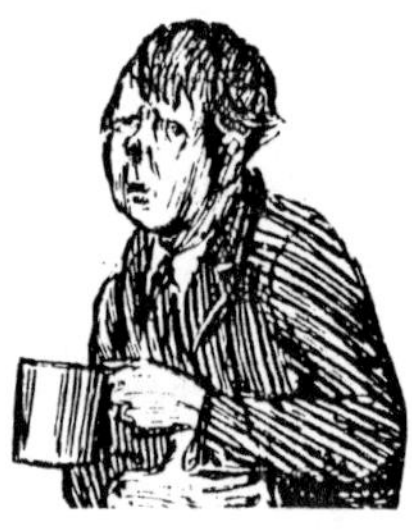

SOCKS 'N ONIONS

Back in the 1930s Doug Langstaff, my grandfather, lived on a small farm near Oakville.

It was during one of those falls in the '30s when Doug fell ill. It all started with a sore throat.

Marion Langstaff, his wife, remembered an old remedy for sore throats.

She cut an onion in two and tied an old dirty and smelly sock around it. Then the smelly sock and the onion were tied around Doug's throat.

After a couple of days, Doug's throat was much improved. At least, he said it was.

My teacher and I have been trying to figure out how that smelly old sock could have done any good for my grandfather. We pretty well decided that the victims of that remedy just pretended to get better to escape another treatment with that awful onion and sock mess.

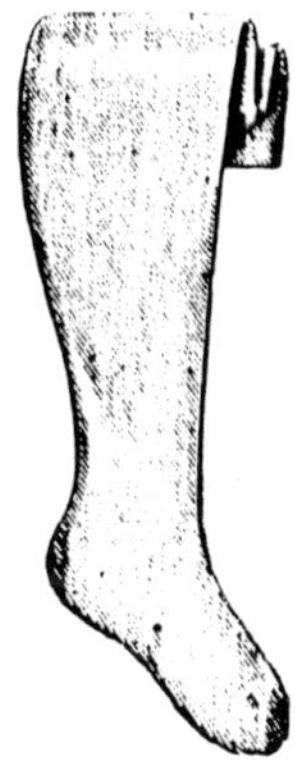

—*by Stephen Brown*

HONEY COMB CHEW

In the 1920s when a cough developed or a scratchy throat came upon a victim, the patient would be given a piece of honeycomb to chew.

Marion Schafer of Wapello remembers that instead of chewing gum or a throat lozenge, his parents would give him a honeycomb to chew on to help a scratchy throat.

Marion said that the honeycomb tasted sweet at first, but it would then lose its taste. However, you had to keep chewing it or you'd get in trouble with your mother.

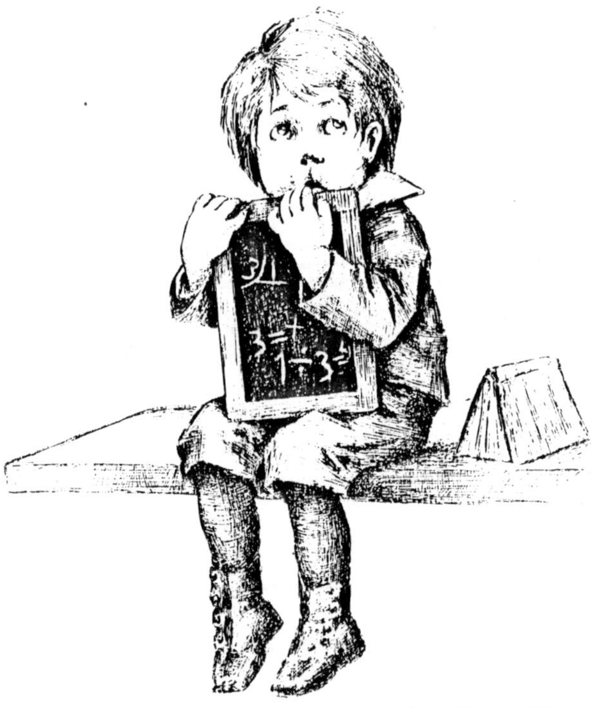

—by Anna Young

SALT WATER TREATMENT

Sylvia Foor of Wapello always had her children gargle salt water when they had a sore throat.

Without fail, if any of the children showed even the slightest hint of a sore throat, out would come the salt water gargle.

It tasted terrible, but it worked, and that's what counted.

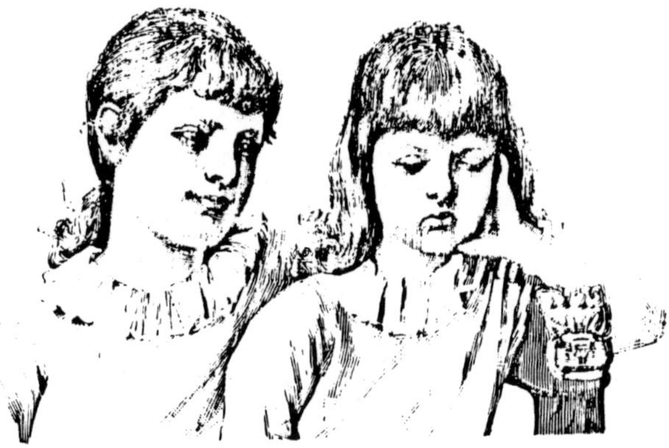

—by Ryan Foor

HICCUPS

Being a family of five, there was often one of us who had the hiccups at one time or the other.

We tried the usual "hold your breath" routine to try to get rid of them, and that didn't work. We tried the "drink a whole glass of water without stopping" trick. That didn't work either.

Then, one day, my stepfather suggested I drink water out of a glass backwards.

At first I thought he was fooling me since he was always doing that, but he said he wasn't. So I asked him how to do it.

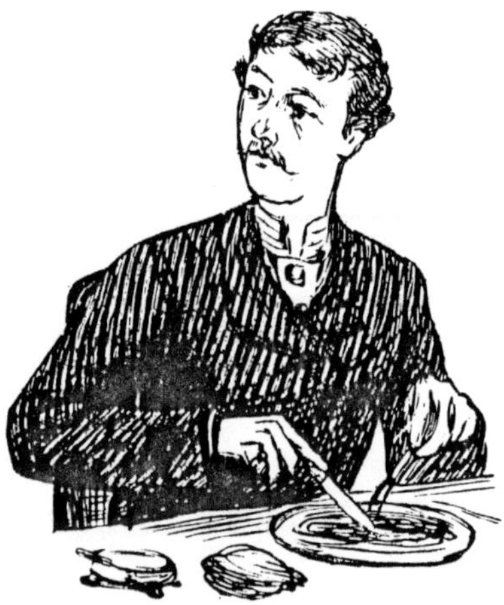

He showed me and it worked. This cure has never failed me.

—by Crystal Housman

POULTICE REMEDIES

BREAD AND MILK POULTICE

Page Kepper grew up in the little town of Winfield.

At that time there weren't any drugstores in town, and the folks didn't go to the doctor unless they just had no alternative.

Folks around Winfield relied on home remedies made from things around the house or in the woods for a lot of their medical problems.

Once Page cut her finger on a thorn. Her mother's care consisted of scalding a little milk and then dipping a piece of bread in the milk until the bread was completely soggy.

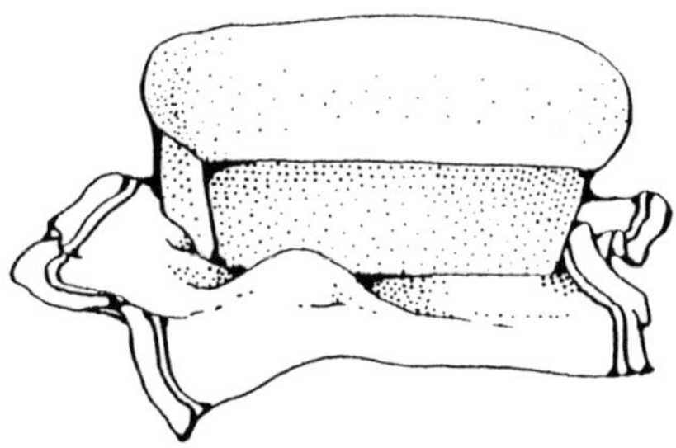

Then Page's mother put the bread over the cut and wrapped it in a bandage. By morning that severely infected cut was clear of infection and felt much better.

—by Les Hollingsworth

CURES FOR A COLD

In the early 1900s my Grandma and Grandpa Fletcher were kids growing up around Columbus Junction.

Their families, like others in the area, used skunk oil and goose grease for their colds.

Their fathers would set traps in the nearby woods and catch those striped critters. In the winter, a skunk has about a half inch of fat next to the hide.

The victims of those traps were skinned, and the fat rendered out.

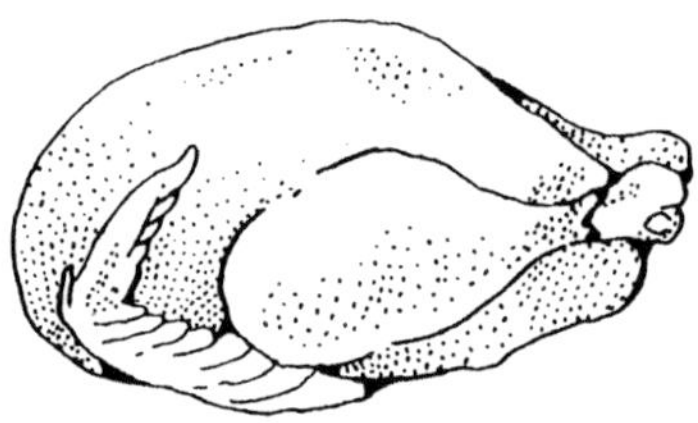

Then, too, many a goose laid down his life for the battle against the common cold also. It was undoubtedly a project for which the goose didn't have a whole lot of enthusium.

—by Daniel Bryant

ONION POULTICE

Sometimes many remedies had to be tried before one "worked". After trying the mustard plaster remedy and not getting any satisfactory results, mothers might try the onion poultice.

This remedy consisted of cooking onions over the old cookstove until tender. They were then applied

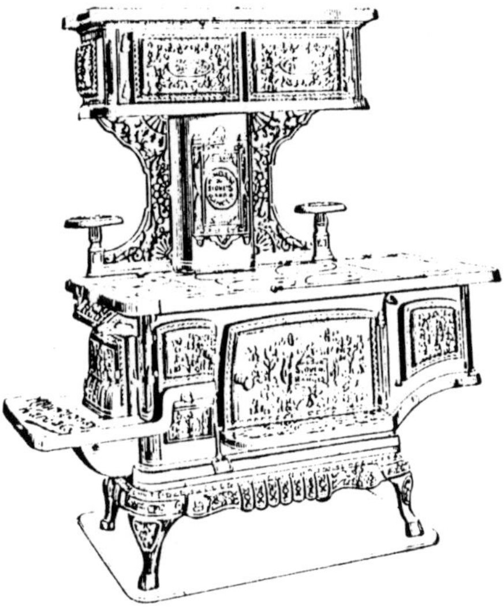

to the chest much like the mustard plaster, after the onions had cooled off enough. This method was usually reserved for the more serious coughs.

There are older folks whose coughs have long since faded, but their memories of those poultices live on.

—by Denise Lanz

MUSTARD PLASTER

Winter always brought its share of colds and bad coughs. Since mothers could not depend on cough syrup or other modern medicines, they developed this remedy to ease the coughing.

Mix two parts flour with one part of dry mustard, and add enough water to make a thick paste.

Spread this paste between two pieces of cloth such as old pillowcases, and put it all on the patient's chest.

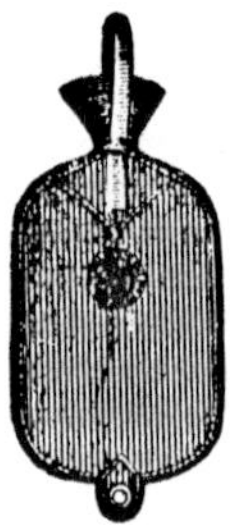

Fill a hot water bottle and put it on top of the mustard plaster secured by bath towels and the blankets snugged in tight around the child's chest.

Every so often, the mother would check to see if the skin had turned pink. When she was satisfied, she'd remove the plaster and rub the chest vigorously with Vicks or Menthoatum. The hot water bottle would be refilled and put back on the chest.

This remedy was usually very reliable, and many mothers still doctor with a good vigorous rub.

—by Denise Lanz

CHEST COLDS

"ACHOOOOOOOO! I hate it when I have a chest cold. Oh well, after another spoonful of icky horrible tasting miracle medicine, I'll feel better."

My great-grandmother, Edna Heater, lived near Columbus Junction in the days they didn't have miracle medicine. When she was a girl, they had no drugstore to go to get medicine for chest colds.

Edna's mother used a remedy made of a mixture of mustard powder with just the right amount of smelly apple cider vinegar. This would make a sticky, pasty mustard plaster. She would spread the plaster on a small cloth, cover it with a stove-warmed larger wool cloth.

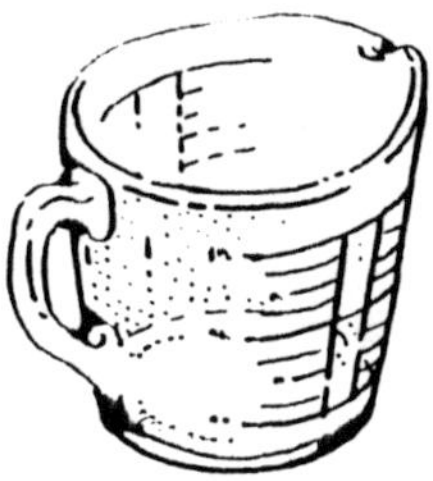

After all that, the whole thing would be slapped on Edna's bare chest and Edna was sent to bed for a good night's sleep. Somehow the remedy eased the chest pain and the coughing.

—by Jaime Heater

PINK SKIN AND EGGS

When Cordell Hagele was growing up on the farm, he as well as many other children had a terrible cough with their colds.

His mother, Minnie, had a solution for the problem. She would mix a tablespoon of flour and a tablespoon of mustard powder with a small amount of water and the beaten white of an egg.

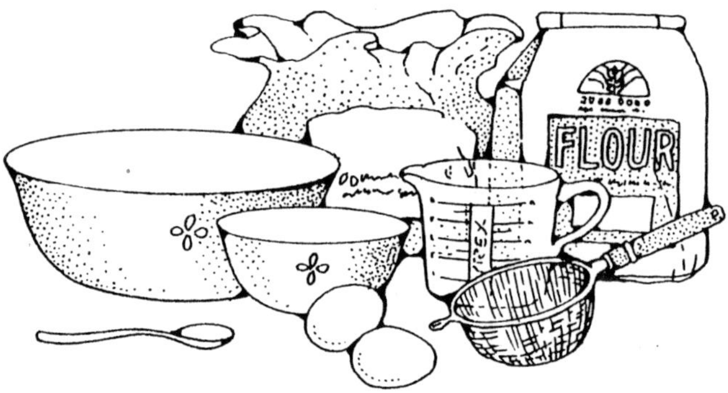

She would leave this on Cordell's chest until Cordell's skin began to turn a red or nice pink color.

She kept the plaster moist in waxed paper, and when the skin turned normal color again, she'd give him another dose of it. Again, the skin would turn red from that plaster.

After this second time, Minnie would put it all away

and keep his chest well covered and warm. That always did the trick and the child would get a good night's rest.

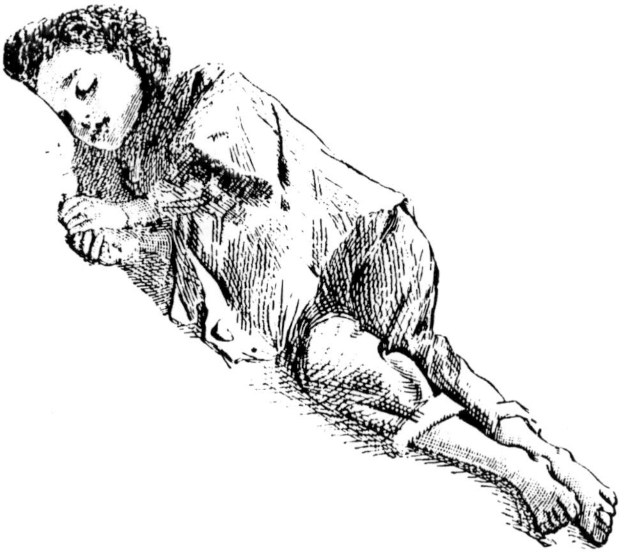

—by Mike Hagele

MINNIE AND MENTHOLATUM

It got downright cold on the Mississippi River in the early 1900s. So when fall came the Hagele family had to have fuel. The father and the eldest son hitched up the horses and headed for the river to get a load of driftwood. They used this driftwood in both the kitchen range and in the potbelly stove in the parlor to keep the house warm.

The father and son sawed the logs into short pieces about a foot long with a two-man hand saw and then split those pieces by hand with axes.

Some of the younger kids carried armloads of this wood to the shanty and stacked it, where it would stay dry, ready for use. Each morning before going to school, and again, after school, one of the children had to bring an armful of wood in for the day and evening.

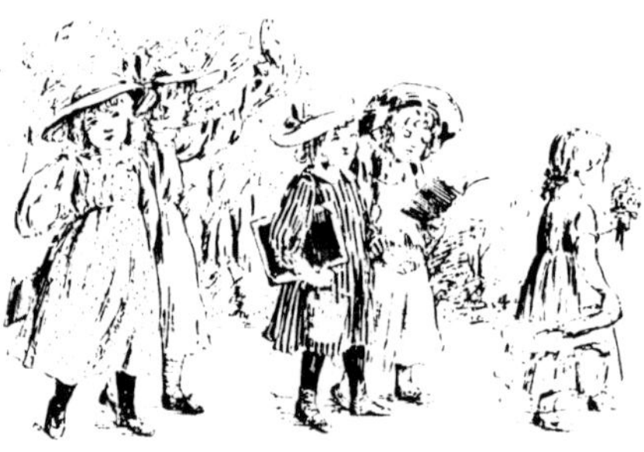

Often, especially during the winter months, the children, first one and then another, would catch a cold and have severe sore throats, many times, even causing earaches.

In those days people seldom went to see a doctor. Instead, they used home remedies.

For some throats, Minnie Hagele would dip a goose feather in warmed alcohol and swab the throats of her children. The children didn't care for that a whole lot because it would make a burning feeling.

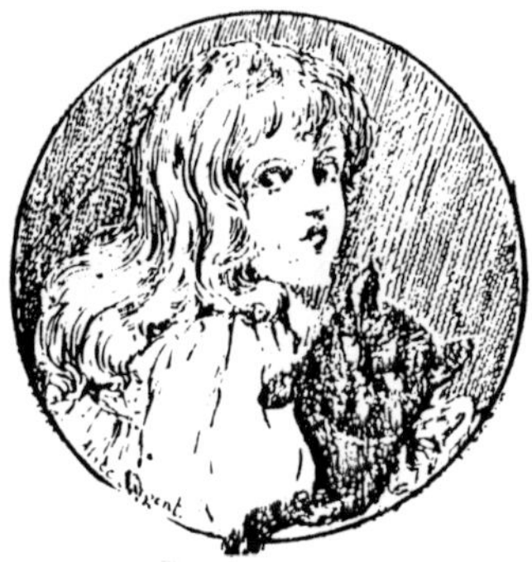

Also, she'd stand behind the child and she'd rub the throat vigorously with Mentholatum or Vicks.

Finally, she'd soak a cotton cloth in cold water and fold it so she could tie it around the throat covering that with a piece of wool to keep the medicine in.

—by Mike Hagele

CHEESE POULTICE

One day in the early 1900s, Ivan Newman became very sick.

He was coughing and his chest hurt when he took the slightest breath and he had a fever. It was decided later that he probably had a bad case of pneumonia.

Ivan's wife, Valeda, remembered an old family remedy. She took some cheese and some potatoes and tried to remember just how to put that old remedy together.

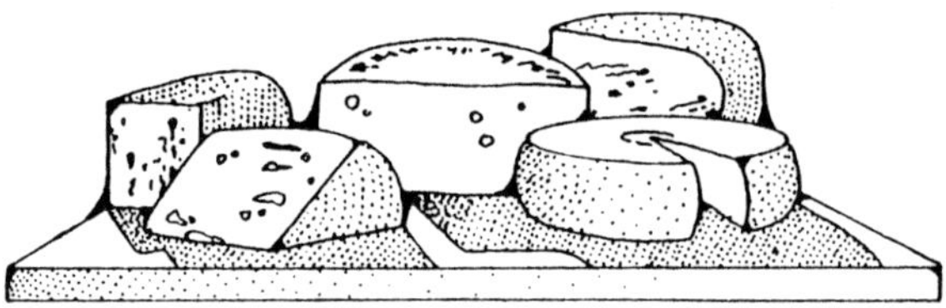

As she remembered her grandmother doing that poultice, it all came back to her. She cut some of that cheese up along with some potatoes and put it all in a cloth before heating it up.

When it was good and hot and the cheese was starting to melt, she put the whole thing on Ivan's chest, and left it there for two days. It worked.

—by Nathan Newman

CHEST COLDS

A chest cold in the early 1900s was often a serious thing and could easily lead to pneumonia.

Money was scarce and people tried to "doctor" themselves as best they could.

Harriette Hanson, who lived by Dubuque, fell victim to a bad chest cold back then.

Her mother was ready for that, though, Harriette's mother rubbed some goose grease onto a cloth and laid that cloth on her daughter's chest. She left it there for a full three hours.

Every now and then Harriette's mother would add more goose grease. This went on for several times, and before the day was out, Harriette felt real good again.

One thing, though, just because the cloth and the goose grease were taken away didn't mean the smell was done. Harriette carried that with her for a while.

—by Nathan Newman

CAMPHOR OIL AND A WOOL CLOTH

One old time remedy for chest congestion was the practice of using camphor oil and a wool cloth.

My grandmother, Laurie Sherry Dorothy, often used this remedy as a child growing up in the Midwest during the depression in the 1930s.

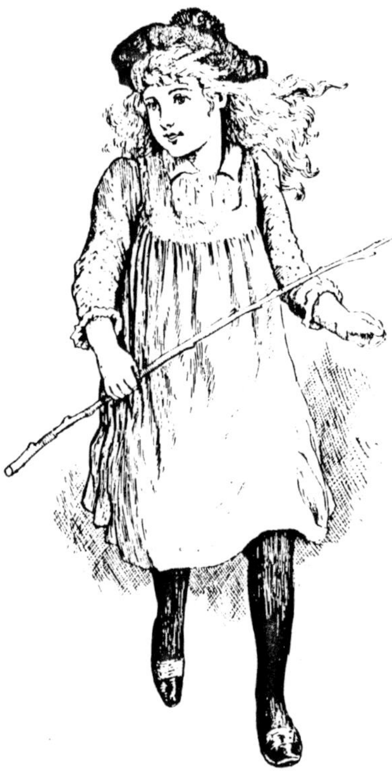

The standard procedure was to apply camphor oil to the skin on the chest, with a wool cloth placed over the chest. A similar procedure was used for a sore throat.

The cloth was left in place all day or even overnight, and often seemed to help reduce the congestion.

When the cloth was removed, the camphor was washed from the skin. Often, however, like Harriette Hanson's good grease, the smell would stay with her for some time.

—by Bob Hodges

WALLPAPER POULTICE

In the early 1900s chest colds often led to pneumonia. Since antibiotics had not yet been developed, pneumonia was very serious. There were remedies and many variations of remedies.

Ivan and Valeda Newman, parents of Mike Newman, who now lives near Wapello were living in a small town near Davenport. Ivan developed a chest cold that turned into pneumonia.

Valeda used a family remedy that had been in the family a long time then already.

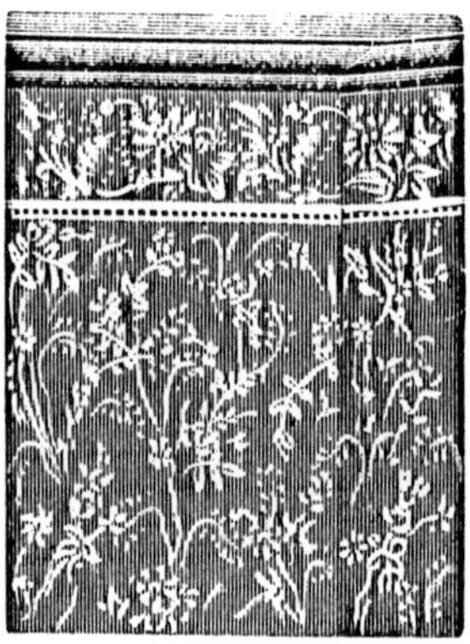

Valeda took a piece of wallpaper right off the wall, and spread some mustard all over that sheet of paper. She then put it on Ivan's chest and heated that paper with a flatiron from the stove. For four days, Valeda kept that up. She had to keep the flat iron warmed all the time and had to keep that stove going for all that time.

After the fourth day, Valeda took the paper off.

Both Valeda and Ivan had a concern about that mustard. Left long enough, that spice could actually damage the skin and leave a bad scar.

But they were willing to run that risk since pneumonia was a lot more serious than a scar.

Ivan emerged unscarred and well again.

—by Nathan Newman

TURPENTINE FOR CHEST COLDS

In the early 1900s, turpentine was a household supply item that very useful. It could be used outside and for internal purposes also. Folks would buy turpentine from the general stores. Every home had a can of it since it had so many uses.

Bub Kreiger from Mt. Union remembers that, as a boy, turpentine was mixed with lard from various farm animals. This mixture was the main cure for chest colds in the Krieger household.

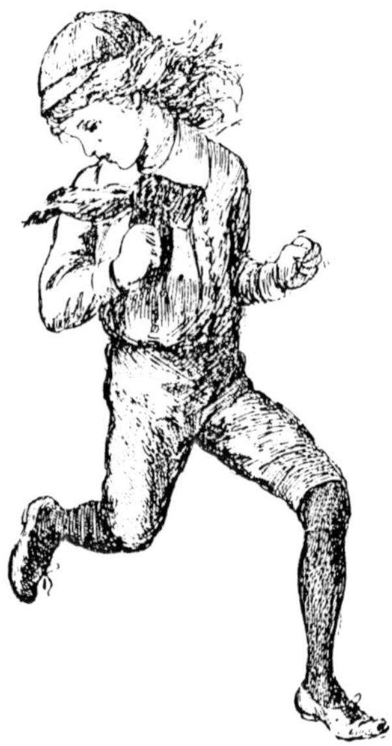

Bub recalls the times, as a young boy, that his father's rough hands would rub the mixture on his skin. That rough treatment was enough to make a boy try not to get a chest cold.

After that rubdown, his father would lay a hot piece of cloth over Bub's chest.

That cloth would have been heated on the cookstove, and then more lard and turpentine would be put on it.

Usually there would be no chest cold left in the morning, only a very red chest.

—by Anna Reighard

GOOSE GREASE

Keith Larson, a former teacher and farmer in Muscatine County, remembers that at holiday time in his childhood, a plump goose was important for several reasons.

The meat, of course, was deliciously prepared and cooked for eating.

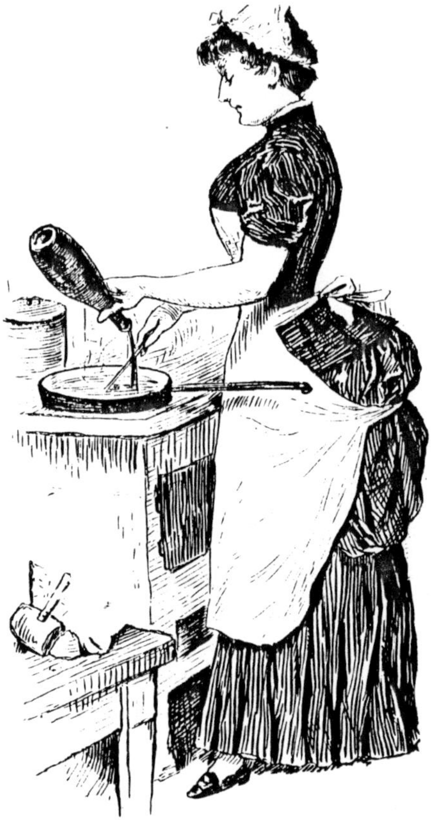

The down was saved for pillows, mattresses, and comforters. And, the fat was carefully preserved in a jar to be used for medical purposes.

Goose grease was rubbed manually on the chest and throat to alleviate sore throat and early symptons of pneumonia. It was also applied to a cloth that had been heated on the oven door of the cook stove, and then wrapped tightly around the neck and worn all day for sore throat.

Sometimes a kid would even be made to wear that cloth to school.

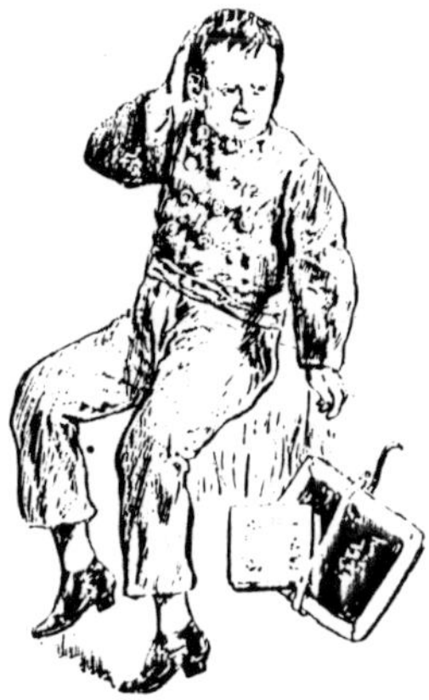

Of course, very often it would come off and hidden in the woods to be put on again when the kid would come back from school.

The combination of the heat and the goose grease was a much respected remedy among parents, of course. Looking back, Keith can still smell those goose grease things he had put on his chest so many times. One wonders what medicinal effects the aroma had on the bronchial tubes.

—by Anna Young

FEVER

During the depression, money was scarce. Ron Cross of Wapello remembers their house being real chilly. Heating a whole house cost too much. The kitchen was the warmest room in the house because of the cookstove, so that's where they would stay most of the time.

Sometimes when it got really, really cold the family would move the beds right into the kitchen.

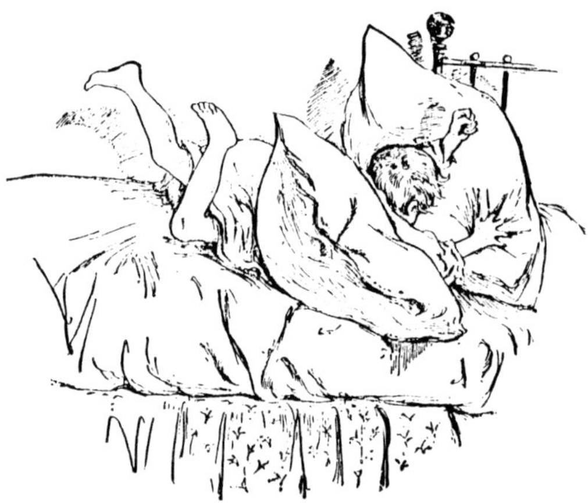

There was something kind of nice about jumping into bed to the sound of the teakettle on the stove.

One time Ron's brother had a very high fever. The family didn't even consider taking the boy to the doctor or to buy medicine. There was no money for that. Home remedies were the only ones available.

Ron's mother took care of his brother that time

with those reliable old home remedies like she had all the other times she had a sick child.

She dipped a cloth in nice warm water, smeared some mustard seeds on the cloth, then placed it on the boy's forehead.

Within just a few minutes the fever was broken, and the boy was on the way to recovery.

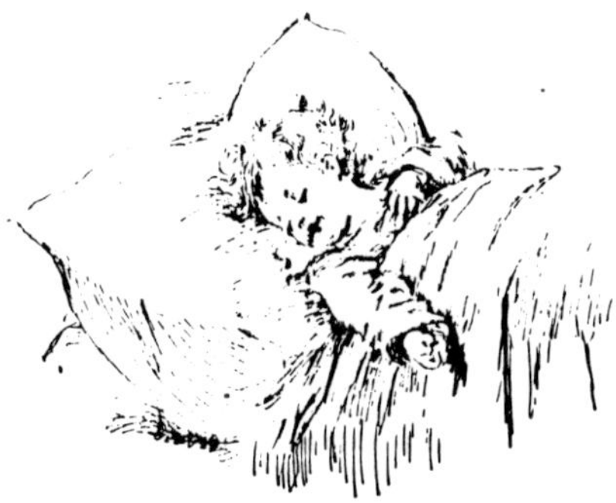

—by Travis Lowe

REMEDIES FOR:

Removal of Thorns and Splinters

BACON AND SPLINTERS

In the early 1900s when Jerry Bean built anything out of wood he would always seem to get some splinters.

Jerry's mother would have him put some bacon on it and tie in fast with a piece of string.

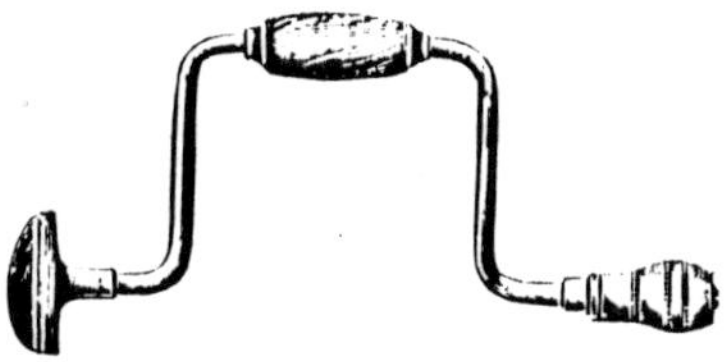

That old splinter would soak up some fat from that piece of bacon and slip right out of that finger like it had been greased.

—by Erin Spitznogle

SPLINTERS

Many years ago when many Iowa men were at war, it was necessary for some of the women to chop the wood to keep the houses warm.

One day Bonnie Dotson went out and no sooner got started chopping some firewood but what she got was a splinter in her finger.

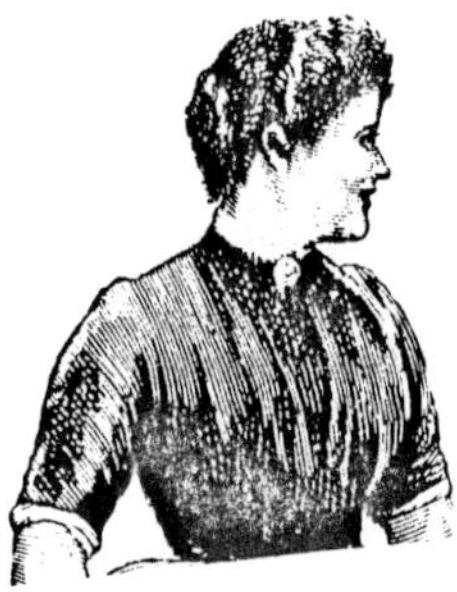

No matter how some other family folks tried to get that splinter out, they just couldn't seem to make it budge.

So Bonnie got a fresh egg from the chicken cook. She took that real fresh egg to the kitchen and broke it open, saving only the shell.

Carefully, Bonnie peeled that soft lining out from the inside of the shell. She laid that lining on the finger with the sliver and it pulled that sliver right out of her finger.

—by Jason Cross

SPLINTER REMOVAL

Carol Rawhouser, my grandmother, lived on a farm most of her life so she learned to use home remedies for medical problems.

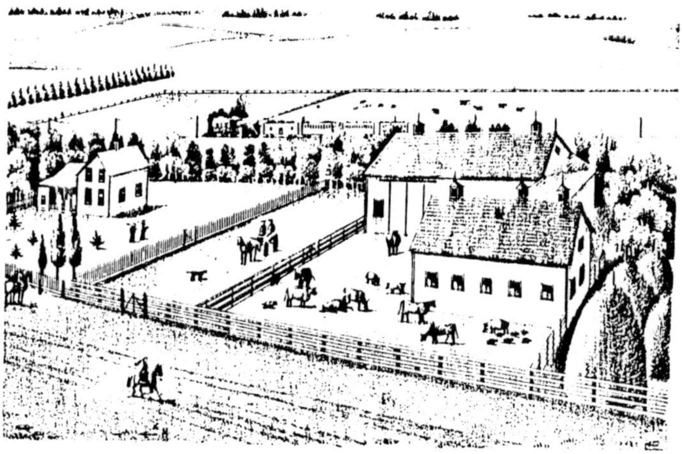

One such remedy was to remove splinters. What she would do is to mix one tablespoon of water with three tablespoons of flour to make a thick paste. That she would apply this to an infection or a splinter and then cover with a bandage for two days.

Once, not too long ago, my father got a bad splinter in his finger and remembered Grandma's remedy. He used it and that sliver was out within two days.

—by Les Hollingsworth

DEW TOE

Gladys McNeil of Louisa County remembers what her mother used to do to treat a condition called "dew toe".

Dew toe is a painful condition in which cracks develop in the joints on the under side of the toe. Apparently it is from going barefooted all summer, which most kids did in the early 1900s.

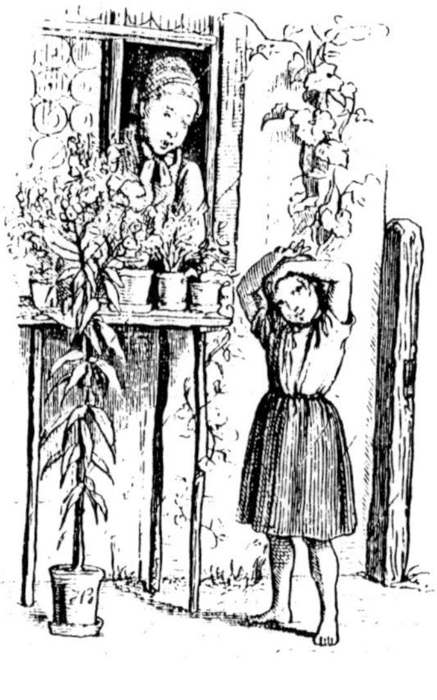

Gladys's mother would tie a string around the toe so it would absorb moisture from the crack. That, in turn, would aid in the healing of the toe.

—by Nichole Simmons

THORN WRAP

When my Grandma Lois Robbins was a young child durring the early 1900s, she would play outside a lot with her older brothers and sisters. Since they lived on a farm, there was plenty for them to do.

Usually, by the end of the day, she or one of her brothers or sisters had a thorn in their hand or foot.

When those children showed up in the house with a thorn, their mother, Pearl, would first try to get it out with one of her sewing needles. If that didn't work, she'd get a little bottle of flax seed out of her cupboard.

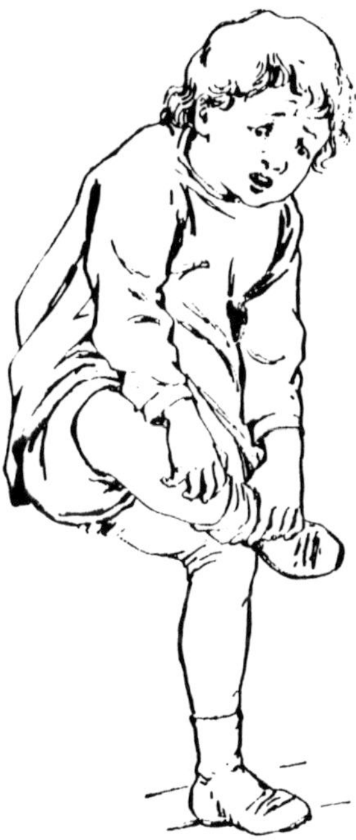

Pearl would smash a few of those seeds with water to make a paste.

She'd put that paste on the skin where that thorn was and cover it with gauze overnight.

—by Crystal Housman

PREVENTIVE PROCEDURES

SPRING TONIC

A spring tonic was always given to Mae Larson's family and many others in a Mississippi River community in the 1920s.

Mae, the pastor's wife, felt the blood became sluggish and polluted during the winter. People were kind of slow moving because their blood was sluggish. So, everyone, children and adults, needed a Spring Tonic.

When the first bud appeared on the apple tree on the first crocus bud broke the cold earth's surface, Mae went to the woods with her three sons to dig sassafrass roots.

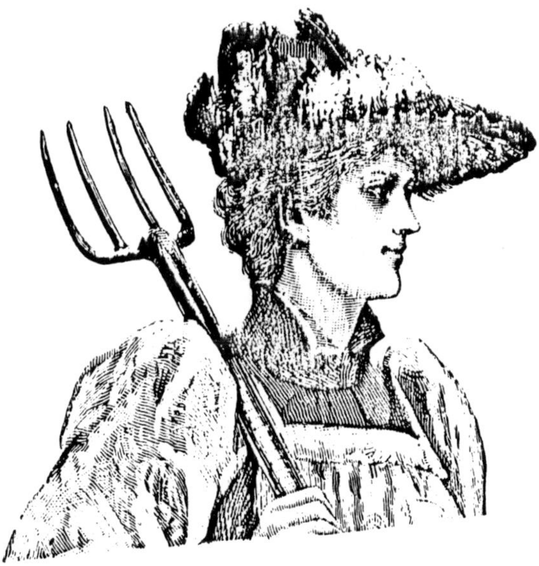

She would then dry those roots, cut them into chunks and grind them up.

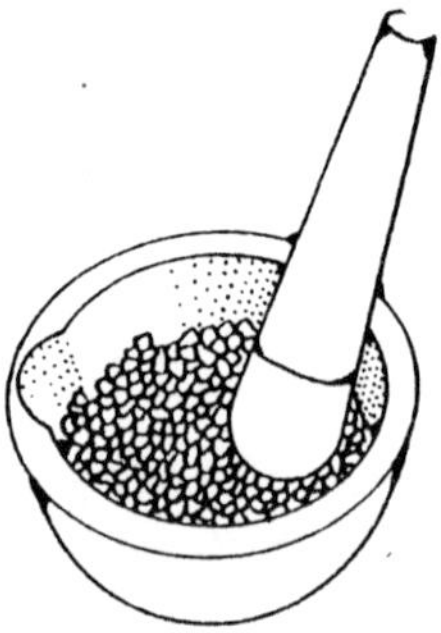

Then for several weeks the whole family would drink a tea that she would make from those roots. That was supposed to give them energy for all the coming work in the spring and summer.

Today we recognize the smell of sassafrass roots as root beer.

It is common knowledge that the Indians here in North America drank sassafrass tea, so maybe that is where the use originated.

Mae Larson's ancestors were some of the first settlers down in Tennessee and would have come in contact with the Indians of that area.

Whether sassafrass tea actually gives a person energy or not for the coming spring remains a matter of opinion, but the smell is wonderful.

—by Anna Young

BUCK-EYES FOR A NECKLACE

Usually we think of the Indians as wearing necklaces with special medicinal effects to prevent sicknesses or to ward off evil. But, our own ancestors, even in the early 1900s, also wore some special preventive necklaces.

One such necklace was from Toller Hayes here along the Mississippi River.

Toller would string a buckeye and tie them into a necklace. He would provide each of his two sons with one of those to wear around their necks to ward off chest ailments.

An interesting experiment to do here in Iowa yet today is to mention buckeyes in a group of farmers in a cafe or at an auction. Almost invariably, one of the fellows will have one on him somewhere in his pockets.

—by Jarett Ball

ASAFETIDA

Crystal Schmeizer remembers that some folks in the early 1900s wore a bad smelling substance in a small bag tied around their neck to ward off illnesses. This was called an asafetida.

The substance in the bag varied. Some wore garlic. The dictionary says the substance was from the Asiatic plants of the parsley family.

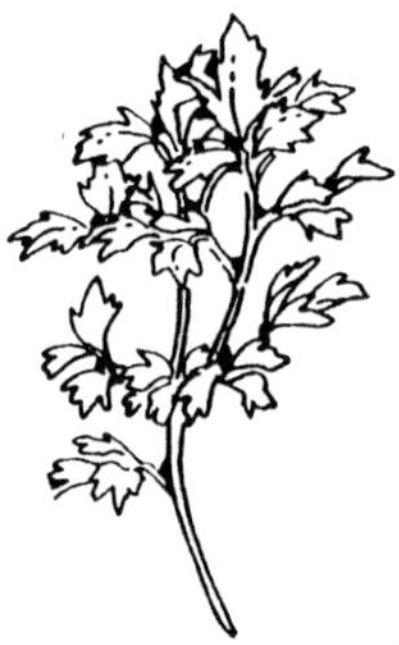

One wonders how something worn around the neck could have been useful. Maybe the smell did do something to the germs.

Another theory is that the smell was often so bad that it kept others at a distance. Maybe it kept folks so far away that the wearer of that smelly little bag didn't get exposed to so many germs.

—by Anna Young

REMEDIES FOR:

Boils

BOILS

A boil is a large pimple-like infection on the body. It is treated by giving the patient antibiotics. And, if it doesn't heal in a reasonable time, the doctor will often lance the boil and remove the core.

Back around the turn of the century, it was not easy to get to a doctor and antibiotics weren't available. So families had their own favorite methods of treating such things.

Walter Swinderman of rural Charleston had his family collect fresh cow manure and put this onto the boil. It was supposed to make the boil come to a head, so it could be opened with a needle. The core of the thing would then "pop" out.

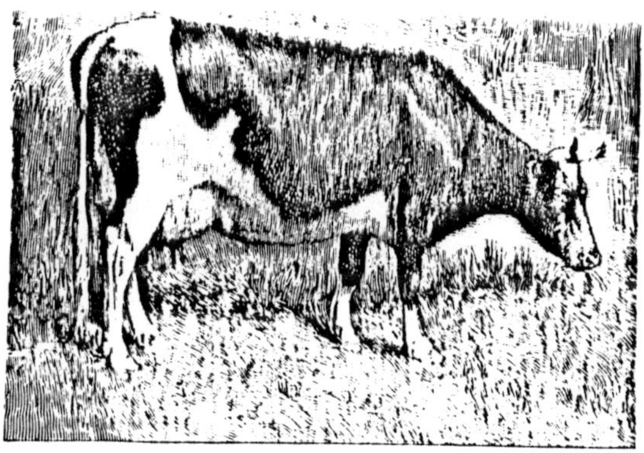

It was important that the cow manure be very fresh so that flies or other insects had not landed on it and laid eggs in it. The idea was . . . the fresher, the better.

I wonder if people went around following after the cow with a pan.

—by Nicole Simmons

BOTTLES FOR BOILS

When Lee Dotson was a little boy growing up on a farm, he would sometimes get infections in his cuts and scrapes.

One time when he got a cut, it became infected. That, in turn, grew into what turned out to be a boil there on his arm.

That boil itched and hurt at the same time. It bothered him a lot, and his arm would throb with the pain of that boil.

But Lee came up with an idea that solved his problem.

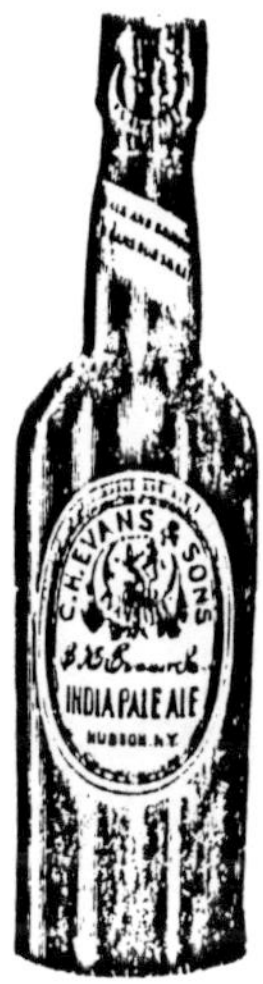

He heated a bottle on the stove until the air inside was good and warm. then he greased the mouth of that bottle and stuck it right on his skin over that boil.

As the air cooled, it made a vaccum and pulled that boil right out of his arm.

Right away his arm felt a lot better, and with the core out of the boil, it healed within just a couple of days.

—by Jason Cross

BOILS

In the days when Carol Rawhouser or one of her children got a boil she would make a home remedy her mother taught her.

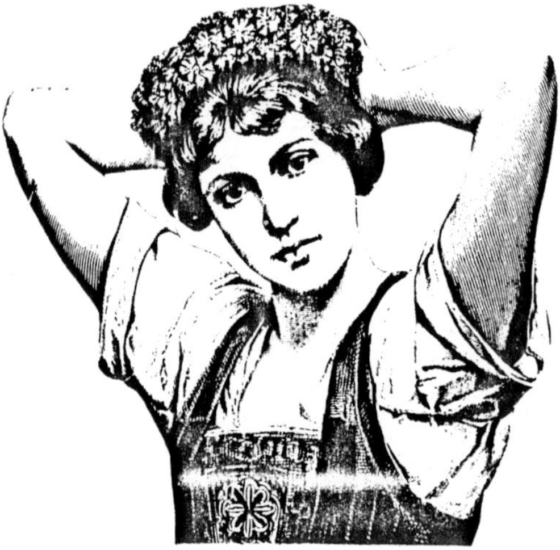

Carol mixed one half a teaspoon of unsalted lard with some flour to make a salve. She would put the mixture over the boil, then wrap it in a bandage.

This would eventually pull the core out of the boil. It would come out so quickly and painlessly that a person could go to sleep with a boil but wake up without one.

—by Les Hollingsworth

FACE THE FACTS, FOR BOILS USE FLAX

In the 1920s people used a lot of remedies because money was scarce and doctors were, too.

On one farm about five miles from Wapello, Orville Schmeiser would, for some reason, often get boils.

Orville's mother would take a handful of flax seed, add water, and heat the mixture until it was thick and soupy.

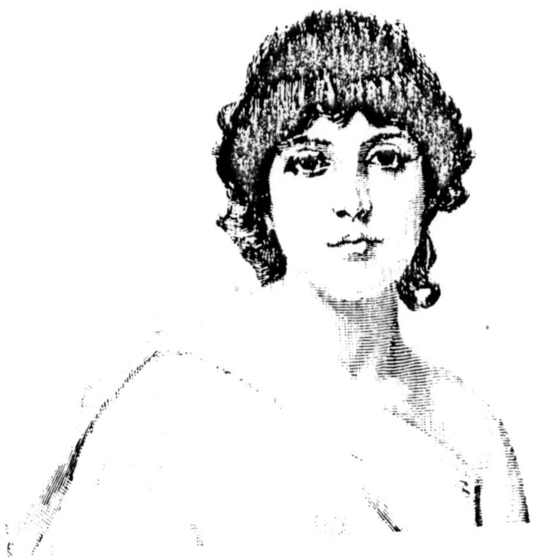

Then she would put the paste to the boil. In a short while, it would be gone.

—by Aaron Locke

REMEDIES FOR:

Coughs
Colds

CHEST PAINS

When chest pains developed, folks around the turn of the century would often fold a slab of salt pork into a piece of sheet or a towel.

They would then put that on their chest, and tie it so it would stay in place.

They would take that off only when they bathed.

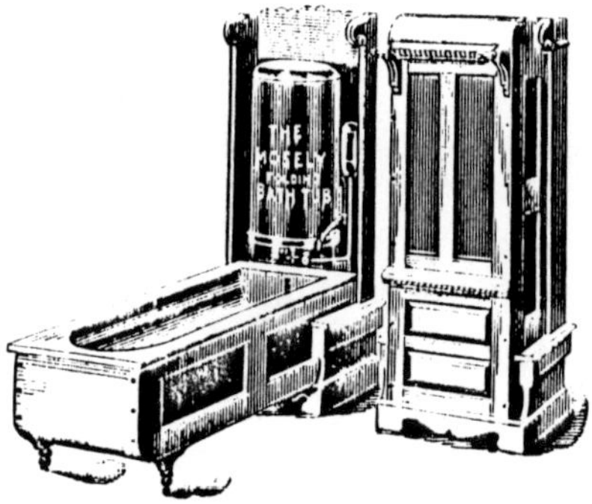

That slab of pork was kept there on the chest until the pain left.

—by Buddy Scott

KATHLEEN AND THE HOREHOUND CANDY

This remedy was helpful in the early 1900s for Kathleen Hagele, the daughter of Raymond and Phyllis McCulley. Many other folks who had bad colds with congestion in the head and chest found this to be helpful, also.

It was a strong horehound candy that did the trick. The honey in the candy also soothed coughs and sore throats. It worked well and worked immediately.

The recipe is:

Horehound Candy

1 ounce fresh horehound or ¼ cup of the dried
1½ cups of water
2 cups of honey
1 cup molasses or black strap molasses

Boil the water in small saucepan. Add horehound and simmer for ten minutes. Allow to stand off the heat for five minutes and then strain liquid into large and heavy 5-quart pot. Add honey and molasses to pot. Mix and cook at medium heat until the temperature slowly reaches the hardcrack stage; 300 to 310 degrees Fahrenheit on a candy thermometer. Scum that forms can be scooped off and thrown away before the candy reaches the high temperature. Do not stir mixture while cooking even though it foams up. Pour into greased 9x13-inch pan and score into pieces before it sets, but as it cools. Mixture will settle and harden as it cools. Refrigerate.

This candy will loosen a stuffed nose and start to bring up phlegm as soon as you put it into your mouth.

—by Mike Hagele

HONEY AND LEMON

My grandmother, Laurie Sherry Dorothy, grew up near Davenport in the 1930s.

Because of the Great Depression of that time, money was in short supply, and doctors and medicines were not as accessible or affordable as now.

When Laurie, as a small girl, caught a cold and a cough, home remedies were often used.

One of those remedies used honey and lemon juice for the treatment of a cough.

Lemon juice, purchased regularly from the local grocery store in the form of canned juice, or, when possible, fresh lemon juice squeezed from lemons, was mixed with the always-on-hand honey.

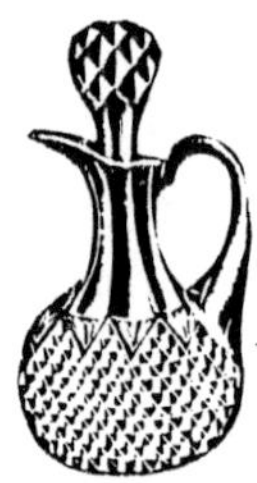

Laurie remembers the mixture usually had more lemon juice than honey, as it remained quite sour.

The concoction was taken orally and seemed to help most times.

—by Bob Hodges

GOOD TASTE FOR A COUGH

My great grandmother, Audrey Ball, lived around the turn of the century back when money was scarce and people had to use what they had. One didn't buy something that you could make yourself.

When anybody got a bad cough, cough syrup from the store was too expensive. Homemade cough remedies were plentiful.

A cough syrup my great grandmother made was a favorite because it tasted great. This was known as Dolly Frank's cough syrup.

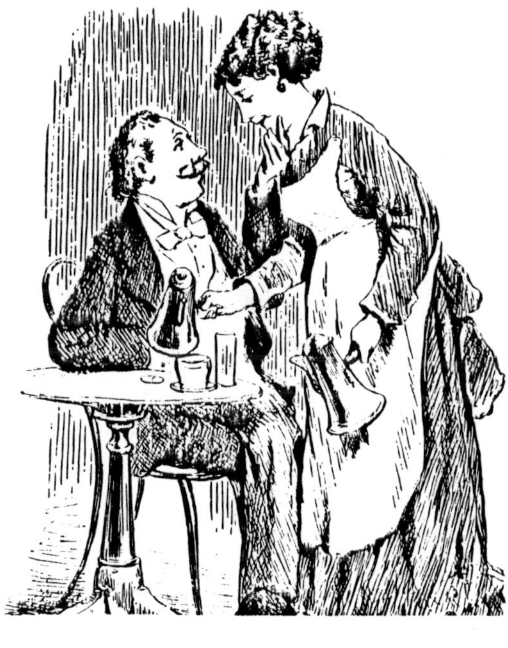

This remedy takes one quart of sugar to two quarts of water. Boil together for twenty-five minutes, then add ten cents worth of powdered rhubarb, and boil again for five minutes. Remove from stove and add ten cents worth of peppermint oil and two tablespoons of soda.

Be sure to use a large pan as it foams up when it settles. Put in a bottle to store.

That cough syrup had such a good taste my great grandmother would have to hide it from the rest of the family.

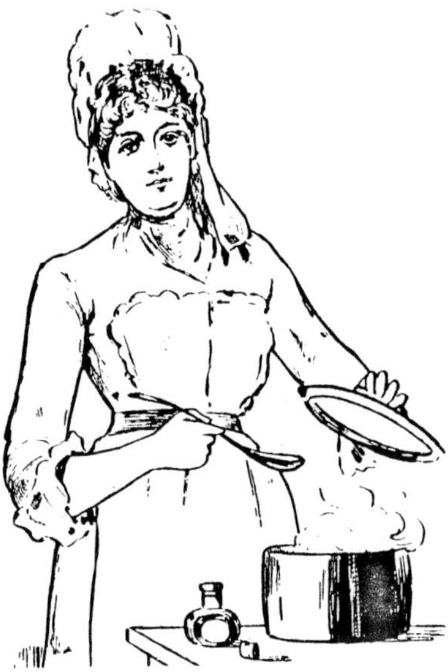

—by Jarett Ball

PLEASE ADD SUGAR

When my grandmother, Heddy Benesh, was young near Ely, there were many remedies for the common cold.

Whenever Heddy or any of her brothers or sisters got sick, their mother would fry an onion in a skillet just until it was transparent. Then she would add some sugar to the onion, cook it a little more, and make a syrup by adding a little water. She would give them a tablespoon of that syrup and tell them to go lie down for a while. I guess that worked, or maybe they just pretended to be well so they wouldn't have to take any more.

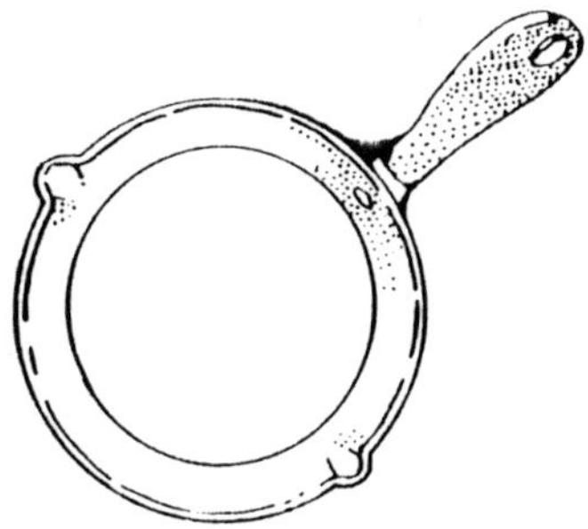

The uncooked version of this cold remedy called for chopping the onion and then putting it in a cloth bag and pounding and squeezing the sucker til it was wet. I'm talking about the onion, not the kid. Then she would add water to the juice and put in enough sugar so the kid's face wouldn't collaspe when he drank it.

—by Tina Samuels

WHAT IS CREOLINE?

About seventy years ago when about three cents would buy a loaf of bread and a dime would get you a gallon of gasoline; doctors were either too far away or too busy to tend to a minor cold. A lot of people had many home remedies for just the common stuffy nose.

One of the most used by Mrs. Orville Schmesier was to heat a dish of creoline on the stove. Then she would put a cloth on her head and lean over the dish. The steam would vaporize the stuffiness and help in breathing.

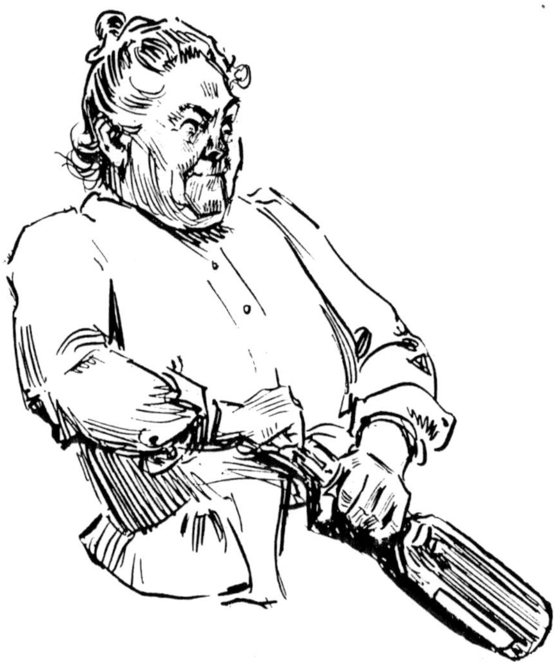

This remedy is more old fashioned than today's electrical vaporizers. I use the electric ones, and I am not sure how the creoline worked.

—by Aaron Locke

P.S. My teacher, Mrs. Young, and I have no idea what creoline is.

A LITTLE BOY AND A STEAM KETTLE

One night many years ago, Lawrence Whipple was sitting in bed with a bad case of congestion. He could hardly move, the felt so bad. Lawrence was only four years old at the time.

His brother said that only twelve people were in school out of eighteen. In a small town like Mediapolis, everybody got sick at the same time.

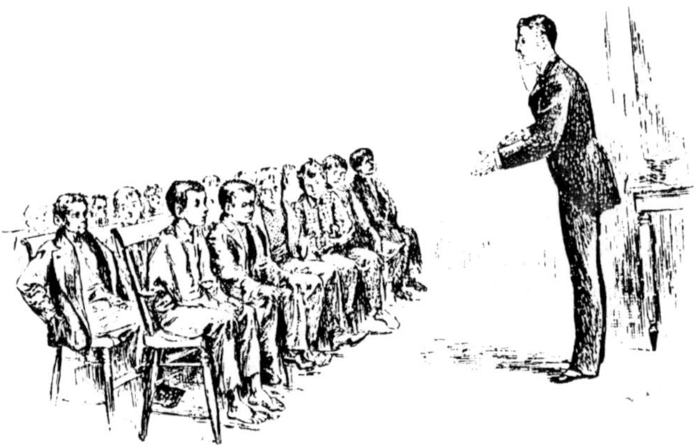

Lawrences's mother had him inhale the steam coming from the tea kettle. He'd carefully take a breath and then back away. He did this several times. Then after a bit he could breathe again. And that's what they did for congestion.

—by Allison Whipple

THE HOT TODDIE

From back in the 1920s, Bub Krieger of Mt. Union remembers his most favorite, but forbidden remedy - the hot toddie.

If Bub had a cold while visiting his grandmother, she would take him into the pantry and get the family whiskey bottle down from the top shelf.

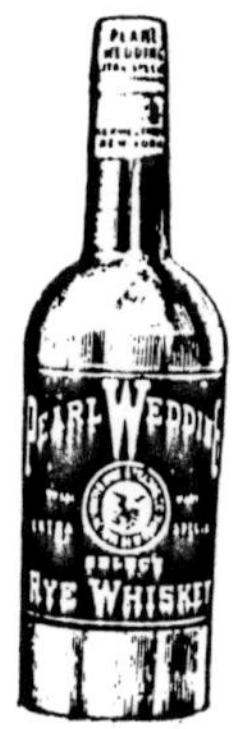

She'd mix a teaspoon of that whiskey with four teaspoons of hot water. These, after a thorough mixing , would be put in a small glass. This hot toddie was a sure cure for colds, coughs, or croup.

Bub thought this was such a delightful cold remedy he would almost always complain of a cold at his grandma's house. Bub enjoyed this hot toddie only until his mother found out what the cure consisted of! That was the end of Grandma's cure.

—by Anna Reighard

REMEDIES FOR:

Infections

KEROSENE FOR ANTISEPTIC

Living on a farm during the depression era presented many problems, especially if there were many children in a family.

Besides the financial problems which always faced a farm family, there was the matter of illness or injury, which forced the parents to treat the patients themselves. Doctors, although very necessary at times, would leave a bill that was very hard to pay. Many mothers learned to be pretty good at doctoring their young. Such was the case of Mary and her family.

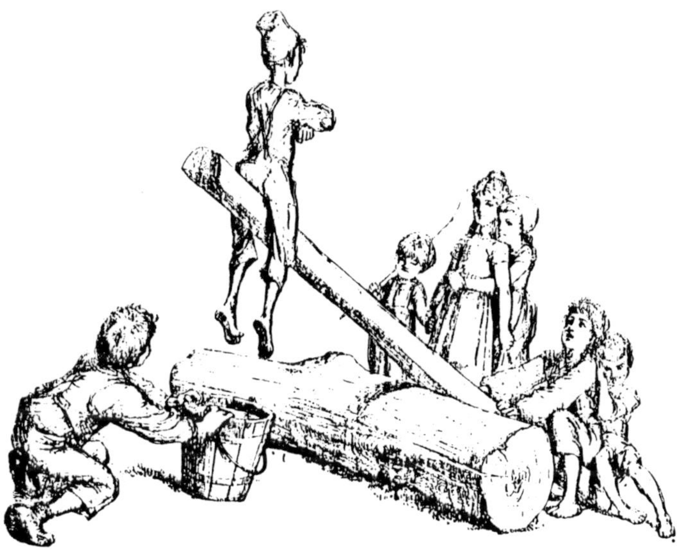

Mary and her husband had five sons and three daughters. As boys can sometimes be very active, one problem seemed to be more chronic than some others. That was stepping on nails that the boys had left lying out from some abandoned project.

Stepping on a nail was often a very painful experience for the victim.

After the nail was removed, Mary would clean out the puncture as best she could. She would then get some kerosene from her kitchen stove and put it in a bucket or tub and have the child soak his foot for about twenty minutes or so. The treatment always seemed to work.

In a time when tetanus was always a possibility, this effective treatment must have been considered to be a good one.

—by Denise Lanz

DANGERS OF GOING BAREFOOT

During the summer months, the Eisenman children had to go barefoot. It simply cost too much to keep eight children in shoes. this wasn't the most pleasant thing - to have to walk barefoot. There were weeds, thistles, little rocks, and sometimes even nails all over the yard.

Once in a while one of the children would step onto a rusty nail. This could, of course, cause infection. So, for a remedy, the foot was soaked in sour milk. This seemed to draw the infection. In those days people just didn't think of going to a doctor for a tetanus shot.

One fall day, two of the girls, Minnie and Elsie, got permission from their parents to go to some friends' house about a mile from home to visit and play with them.

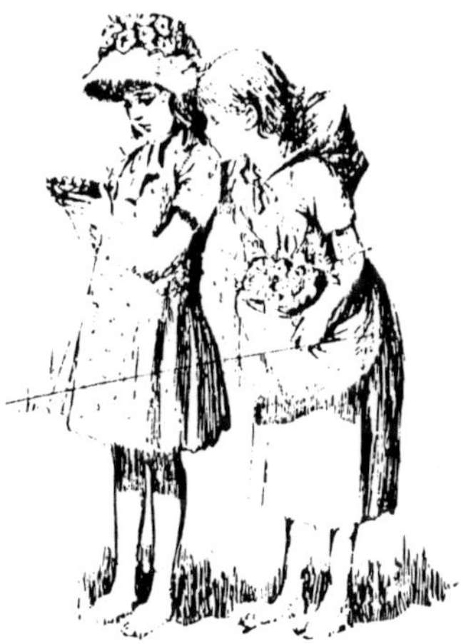

The way was weedy, and while walking along, Elsie felt a sharp prick on the top of her foot. When she looked down, she knew she had been bitten by a small rattler. She saw him slither off into the grass. Two little marks from the fangs confirmed that.

The neighbor was one who chewed tobacco, and after a tourniquet had been put around her leg, the neighbor sucked the poison out of her foot. The tobacco saliva also served as a remedy to fight infection for the time being. He then rode horseback to Elsie's parents place to tell them what had happened.

Within a real short time, the girls' older brother, Albert, came in a car to take Elsie to the doctor, about eight miles away.

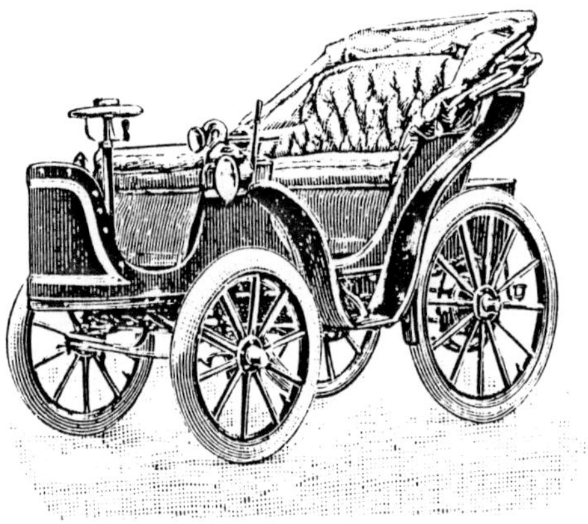

The doctor gave her a shot of serum which was supposed to counteract the venom.

Poor Elsie had to stay home from school for two weeks, keeping her leg elevated. It was badly swollen, all the way to the hip. It was also discolored, a bluish green, like any bruised limb.

The venom of a young rattlesnake was believed to be much more poisonous that that of an older snake. If these home remedies, along with the doctor's care, hadn't been used, Elsie probably would have died.

—by Matt Hagele

THOSE BAREFOOT DAYS

Aunt Rachel Larson, in those early days of the 20th century was a nurse and a doctor combined. The Larsons lived at the Methodist Parsonage. Caleb Larson was the pastor. His children went barefoot all summer and often stubbed big toes on rocks and hay field stubbles.

Aunt Rachel's treatment was a poultice of fat rind and turpentine, well soaked and wrapped with cloth.

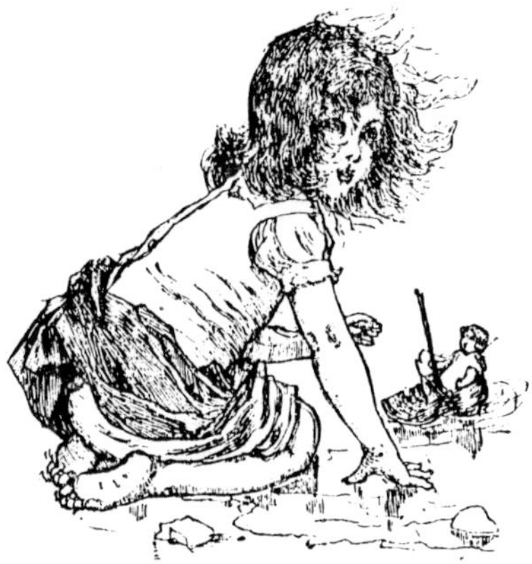

Somehow the poultice always seemed to take away the soreness and was just the right thing for sore toes. Maybe today's Band-Aids and salve does the trick too, but a bandage on a toe felt so comforting.

—by Anna Young

A REMEDY FROM THE FAMILY COWS

Vivian Edmund (Bub) Kreiger was born five miles west of Mt. Union.

Bub was a very active child. He enjoyed riding his pony Billy, playing with his dog, and with his friend, Victor.

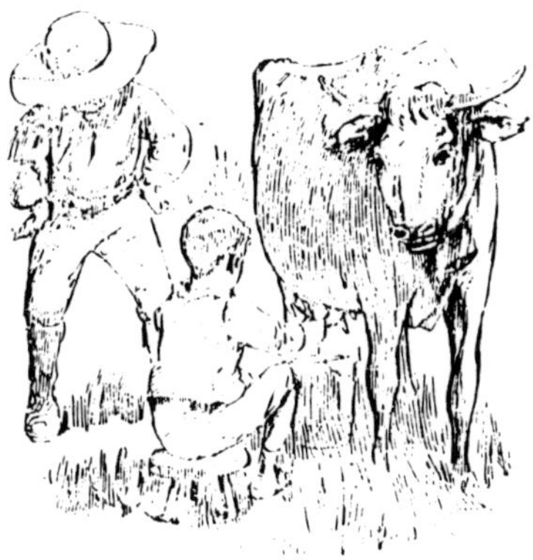

Often, while playing, Bub would step on a nail. Those old rusty nails would easily puncture his skin.

When that would happen, his father would run out to the pasture where the cows were grazing and gather up some fresh manure.

That stuff would be stuck in a gunny sack, and the sack then put over Bob's foot. He would wear that sack like a giant but awful sock. He'd have to drag that thing around for several hours before his parents would let him take it off so they would pour some kerosene onto the wound.

That awful sack would then be replaced by a clean rag wrapped around the foot.

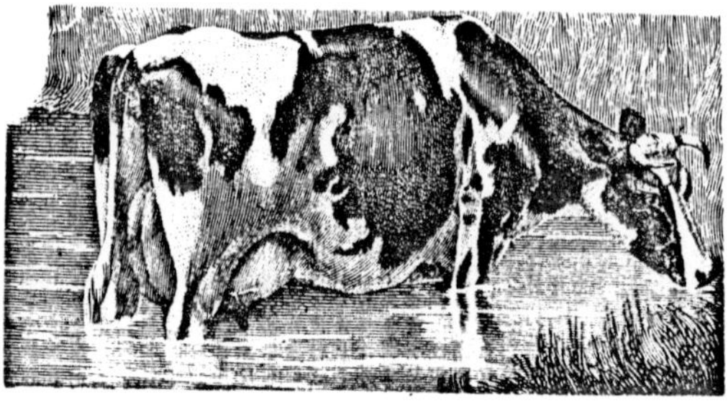

—by Anna Reighard

BEEF FOOT

In the early 1900s, an infection was serious because there were no antibiotics. Home remedies were used and were shared.

Leroy Hanson was living in Dubuque when he stepped on a nail. It went right through his thin shoe and was stuck right in his foot.

Leroy figured his foot would become infected since the nail was old and dirty. So he took a piece of steak and put it right there on the puncture, trying it in place with a piece of cloth.

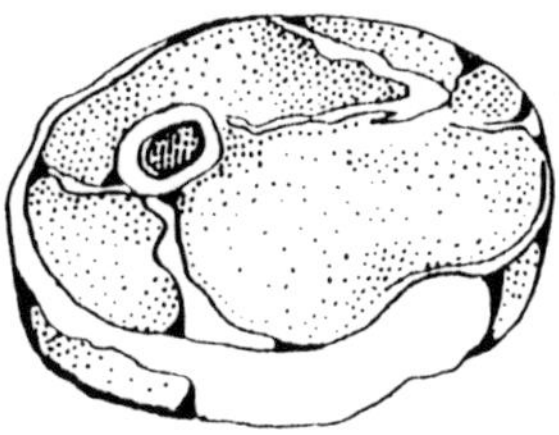

Leroy hobbled around with that piece of steak on his foot for twenty-four hours. After that period of time, he found that the foot felt real good, apparently cured by the steak drawing the poison out of the foot.

—by Nathan Newman

EGGSHELL FOR FELONS

Once in a while, years ago, in Columbus Junction, Lois Bliven would get felons.

Felons are very painful infections near the fingernail or toenail.

Lois would usually get them in the winter. And it was one winter when she got an exremely painful felon on the thumb of her right hand. When she showed that to her parents, her mother had her break open a raw egg.

Her mother took the inside skin of the eggshell and rubbed it on the felon for a time. This cured the felon in a few hours.

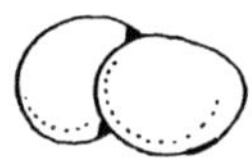

Apparently the eggshell skin drew the infection right out of the felon.

—by Erin Spitznogle

MILK AND BREAD FOR INFECTIONS

An interesting way to draw out an infection came from Mrs. Orville Schmeiser of rural Wapello. She would use a combination of warm milk and bread, and apply this thick soupy mixture to the infected part of the body. It would then set for a time.

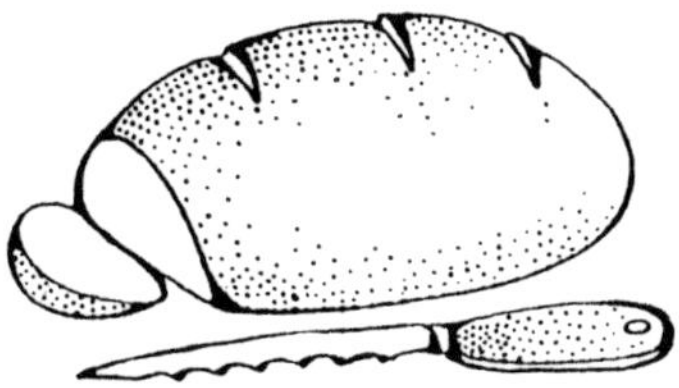

After the paste was removed, the infection would be drawn right out of the wound and the pain would be gone.

—by Aaron Locke

EPILOGUE

All those funny sounding things like skunk oil, creoline, and sweet oil are not used much any more these days in the 1990s. Nor do we think in terms of kerosene, pork rinds, or egg shell liners as being of medicinal value.

But folks back around the turn of the century used those words often and considered them to be important parts of their health care.

While the practice of medicine has changed, the love and care offered to children by their parents are still with us. But then, after all, that's a whole lot more important than goose grease or castor oil.

Need A Gift?

For

• Shower • Birthday • Mother's Day •
• Anniversary • Christmas •

Turn Page for Order Form
(Order Now While Supply Lasts!)

To Order Copies Of

Iowa's Early Home Remedies

Please send me _____ copies of **Iowa's Early Home Remedies** at $9.95 each. (Make checks payable to **QUIXOTE PRESS.**)

Name ______________________________

Street ______________________________

City ______________ State ______ Zip ______

Send Orders To:
Quixote Press
R.R. #4, Box 33B • Blvd. Station
Sioux City, Iowa 51109

- -

To Order Copies Of

Iowa's Early Home Remedies

Please send me _____ copies of **Iowa's Early Home Remedies** at $9.95 each. (Make checks payable to **QUIXOTE PRESS.**)

Name ______________________________

Street ______________________________

City ______________ State ______ Zip ______

Send Orders To:
Quixote Press
R.R. #4, Box 33B • Blvd. Station
Sioux City, Iowa 51109

If you have enjoyed this book, perhaps you would enjoy others from Quixote Press.

GHOSTS OF THE MISSISSIPPI RIVER
Mpls. to Dubuque by Bruce Carlson ....paperback $9.95

GHOSTS OF THE MISSISSIPPI RIVER
Dubuque to Keokuk by Bruce Carlson .....paperback $9.95

GHOSTS OF THE MISSISSIPPI RIVER
Keokuk to St. Louis by Bruce Carlson .....paperback $9.95

GHOSTS OF JOHNSON COUNTY, IOWA
by Lori Erickson ....hardback $12.95

HOW TO TALK MIDWESTERN
by Robert Thomas ....paperback $7.95

GHOSTS OF DES MOINES COUNTY, IOWA
by Bruce Carlson ....hardback $12.00

GHOSTS OF SCOTT COUNTY, IOWA
by Bruce Carlson ....hardback $12.95

GHOSTS OF ROCK ISLAND COUNTY, ILLINOIS
by Bruce Carlson ....hardback $12.95

GHOSTS OF THE AMANA COLONIES
by Lori Erickson......................paperback $9.95

GHOSTS OF NORTHEAST IOWA
by Ruth Hein and Vicky Hinsenbrock .....paperback $9.95

GHOSTS OF POLK COUNTY, IOWA
by Tom Welch........................paperback $9.95

GHOSTS OF THE IOWA GREAT LAKES
by Bruce Carlson......................paperback $9.95

MEMOIRS OF A DAKOTA HUNTER
by Gary Scholl........................paperback $9.95

LOST AND BURIED TREASURE ALONG THE MISSISSIPPI
by Gary Scholl and Netha Bell ....paperback $7.95

(Continued on Next Page)

MISSISSIPPI RIVER PO' FOLK
by Pat Wallace . . . . paperback $9.95

STRANGE FOLKS ALONG THE MISSISSIPPI
by Pat Wallace . . . . paperback $9.95

THE VANISHING OUTHOUSE OF IOWA
by Bruce Carlson . . . . paperback $9.95

THE VANISHING OUTHOUSE OF ILLINOIS
by Bruce Carlson . . . . paperback $9.95

THE VANISHING OUTHOUSE OF MINNESOTA
by Bruce Carlson . . . . paperback $9.95

THE VANISHING OUTHOUSE OF WISCONSIN
by Bruce Carlson . . . . paperback $9.95

MISSISSIPPI RIVER COOKIN' BOOK
by Bruce Carlson . . . . paperback $11.95

IOWA'S ROAD KILL COOKBOOK
by Bruce Carlson . . . . paperback $7.95

HITCH HIKING THE UPPER MIDWEST
by Bruce Carlson . . . . paperback $7.95

IOWA, THE LAND BETWEEN THE VOWELS
by Bruce Carlson . . . . paperback $9.95
(Farm Boy Stories From the Early 1900's)

GHOSTS OF SOUTHWEST MINNESOTA
by Ruth Hein . . . . paperback $9.95

GHOSTS OF THE COAST OF MAINE
by Carole Olivieri Schulte . . . . paperback $9.95

ME 'N WESLEY
by Bruce Carlson . . . . paperback $9.95
(Stories about the homemade toys that farm children made and played with around the turn of the century.)

SOUTH DAKOTA ROAD KILL COOKBOOK
by Bruce Carlson .... paperback $7.95

GHOSTS OF THE BLACK HILLS
by Tom Welch........................... paperback $9.95

Some Pretty Tame, But Kinda Funny Stories About Early DAKOTA LADIES-OF-THE-EVENING
by Tom Welch........................... paperback $9.95

Some Pretty Tame, But Kinda Funny Stories About Early IOWA LADIES-OF-THE EVENING
by Bruce Carlson .... paperback $9.95

Some Pretty Tame, But Kinda Funny Stories About Early ILLINOIS LADIES-OF-THE-EVENING
by Bruce Carlson .... paperback $9.95

Some Pretty Tame, But Kinda Funny Stories About Early MINNESOTA LADIES-OF-THE-EVENING
by Bruce Carlson .... paperback $9.95

Some Pretty Tame, But Kinda Funny Stories About Early WISCONSIN LADIES-OF-THE-EVENING
by Bruce Carlson .... paperback $9.95

Some Pretty Tame, But Kinda Funny Stories About Early MISSOURI LADIES-OF-THE-EVENING
by Bruce Carlson .... paperback $9.95

THE DAKOTA'S VANISHING OUTHOUSE
Bruce Carlson .... paperback $9.95

ILLINOIS' ROAD KILL COOKBOOK
by Bruce Carlson .... paperback $7.95

OLD IOWA HOUSES, YOUNG LOVES
by Bruce Carlson .... paperback $9.95
(Stores about old houses in Iowa and young loves they have known.)

TERROR IN THE BLACK HILLS

by Dick Kennedy .... paperback $9.95

IOWA'S EARLY HOME REMEDIES

by 26 students at Wapello Elem. School ... paperback $9.95

INDEX

INDEX